T0372322

The Spirit of Shiatsu

of related interest

Shiatsu Theory and Practice
Carola Beresford-Cooke
Foreword by Thomas Myers
ISBN 978 1 83997 530 1
eISBN 978 1 78775 845 2

The Extended Meridians of Zen Shiatsu
A Guidebook and Colouring Book
Elaine Liechti and Vicky Smyth
Foreword by Carola Beresford-Cooke
ISBN 978 1 84819 319 2

Working with Death and Loss in Shiatsu Practice
A Guide to Holistic Bodywork in Palliative Care
Tamsin Grainger
Foreword by Richard Reoch
ISBN 978 1 78775 269 6
eISBN 978 1 78775 270 2

The Spirit
of Shiatsu

Ivan Bel

*Forewords by Chris McAlister, Bill Palmer
and Bernard Bouheret*

Translated by Abigail Maneché

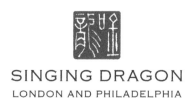

SINGING DRAGON
LONDON AND PHILADELPHIA

First edition published in France in 2022 by Chariot d'Or editions
Part of the Piktos editorial group

First published in English language in Great Britain in 2025 by
Singing Dragon, an imprint of Jessica Kingsley Publishers
Part of John Murray Press

2

Copyright © Ivan Bel 2022, 2025

The right of Ivan Bel to be identified as the Author of the Work has been asserted
by him in accordance with the Copyright, Designs and Patents Act 1988.

Foreword 1 copyright © Bernard Bouheret 2022, 2025
Foreword 2 copyright © Bill Palmer 2025
Foreword 3 copyright © Chris McAlister 2025

Translated by Abigail Maneché

Drawings and computer graphics: Amélie Manchoulas, amypiou.
com, @amypiou, Behance: amypiou unless otherwise stated

Images on pages 72, 73, 203, 277, 283, 284, 286: Adobe.stock.com

Front cover image source: Shutterstock®.

All rights reserved. No part of this publication may be reproduced, stored
in a retrieval system, or transmitted, in any form or by any means without
the prior written permission of the publisher, nor be otherwise circulated
in any form of binding or cover other than that in which it is published and
without a similar condition being imposed on the subsequent purchaser.

A CIP catalogue record for this title is available from the
British Library and the Library of Congress

ISBN 978 1 83997 897 5
eISBN 978 1 83997 898 2

Printed and bound in the United States by Integrated Books International

Jessica Kingsley Publishers' policy is to use papers that are natural,
renewable and recyclable products and made from wood grown in
sustainable forests. The logging and manufacturing processes are expected
to conform to the environmental regulations of the country of origin.

Singing Dragon
Carmelite House
50 Victoria Embankment
London EC4Y 0DZ
www.singingdragon.com

John Murray Press
Part of Hodder & Stoughton Limited
An Hachette UK Company

The authorised representative in the EEA is Hachette Ireland,
8 Castlecourt Centre, Dublin 15, D15 XTP3, Ireland (email: info@hbgi.ie)

Contents

Man: Advanced Principles and Concepts

Heaven: Philosophical Principles and Explanations

Foreword

by Bernard Bouheret

I n this unique and very complete book, Ivan Bel has magnificently succeeded in synthesizing the foundations of Shiatsu and the technical but also spiritual base on which it is built.

He includes, just as in the martial arts that he knows well, the notions of distance, depth, intensity and correct timing. Everything that makes this discipline an art and, also, a Way. Yes, Shiatsu has a Spirit, an invisible frame that underlies its action and penetrates the most closed bodies and hearts.

All sincere practitioners feel invested with this strength.

From the first moments of the session, the patient is asked to remove his shoes and finery, watches, jewels and belt, but to remain dressed, because for the East, only the "Body of Breath", where the Ki circulates, counts and not the body of flesh, bones and blood which are coarse materials. The body of Man is the abode of the Breaths. Then he lies on a futon, on the ground, and the practitioner comes to the same level as him, both then united by Mother Earth with whom he makes an alliance, to root himself in his postures and thus find his strength and balance.

And then comes the rhythm with which he will bathe the body, like a vast swell that carries away all the miasmas, all the impurities, all the stagnations, all the painful memories of which the body is the heavy library.

And the heart is washed! The mind is calmed, and the body restored. Then Life returns.

It all starts with the heart, as the *Su Wen*, the bible of Chinese doctors, points out. If the heart is not peaceful, no treatment will be sustainable. *Shiatsu no kokoro, hahagokoro*: "The heart of Shiatsu is like the heart of a mother" says the Japanese master Namikoshi, and it's so true!

Benevolence, consideration, restraint, all this is expressed in the "Feather Hand" emanating from the "Body of Breath". The hand of the Shiatsu practitioner seeks to soothe the Heart and strengthen the Kidneys, to put the person back in his vertical axis, between Heaven and Earth, between here and now. He must work on his posture for a long time, know how to touch accurately, place his hands skilfully and exert pressure with presence and strength but without brutality. It takes many years of practice to touch the depth of this discipline. Ivan Bel explains the fundamental principles here with great erudition.

Introduced in Europe in the 1960s–70s by Zen monks and Aikidō masters, Shiatsu made its way and continues to take its rightful place alongside alternative medicines, recognized as worthy of interest by the European Parliament in 1997.

Shiatsu is acknowledged in Japan and in 1955 was recognized by its government as a therapeutic discipline. For many years it grew from Chinese medicine (5th–6th century CE) before being developed and refined as a complete energy technique. The Japanese undoubtedly put their mark on it.

The hand goes straight to the essentials, it is performed on the ground; with knees bent one cannot become proud. As such, it is powerful, rhythmic and precise; the deep pressure follows a protocol (*kata*) to restore the free flow of Ki (energy) in the body. It can prevent, treat, improve any disorder that threatens the balance of the being.

Shiatsu is now performed in many practices around the world, but it also has its place in hospitals, and little by little the medical world is getting to know and recognize it.

We wanted to render this aspect in a documentary (*La Voie du Shiatsu*),[1] in which Ivan Bel, other practitioners and I testify, and an accompanying book.[2] In them, we see this manual Japanese medicine radiate in the martial arts community, in hospices, addiction centres, prisons and in the world of art. In the Peruvian mountains, an association has even used it as a tool of non-violence. Shiatsu is a vector of peace, it brings peace to the body and the heart, and it is disarming by its simplicity and ease of approach.

A mat on the floor, a cushion under the knees and the meeting can take place.

I began this practice in 1977 with the fabulous opening of consciousness movement that animated the West at that time. Then, in 1981, I went to train in Kōhō Shiatsu, directly at the source in Japan, in the dojo of its founder (Okuyama Sensei, in Omiya, in the province of Saitama). I lived in the house of the founding master in total immersion, and I was introduced to this therapeutic art as well as Japanese martial practices. Back in France I was no longer the same man, an initiation had taken place—a door had opened forever; a force was connected forever.

I remember the time when, with Hervé Scala (who died in 2015), companion of the Way with whom we had created a dojo in 1982 in Montpellier, we admired and were very surprised by the effects that Shiatsu could have. There was after each treatment a lightness, an intense vibration, a dilation of the heart and a deep feeling of joy that animated the whole body and that no other technique had ever given us. Neither massage, nor acupuncture, nor osteopathy (that we had received from very distinguished hands) had given us such a feeling. And we then asked ourselves: How can Shiatsu do this? What is its *modus operandi?* How to explain it? Where's the secret?

In fact, Shiatsu can be lived in different aspects:

First is a preventive aspect, often practised daily within a family, between its different members. Children may give Shiatsu on the shoulders of their elders and receive a small coin in return. The husband can offer it to his wife and vice versa. The mother or father can watch over the health of their children every day and often avoid a doctor's visit. That's what I did for my three children, and my granddaughter received care on the second day after she was born. What a joy to be able to work with your hands alone!

First is a therapeutic aspect can be provided by qualified and seasoned practitioners who can do a health assessment and regulate the major rhythms of the body. This Shiatsu has many beneficial effects for numerous modern disorders such as: insomnia, colitis, muscle pain, lumbago, headaches, depression, fatigue, etc. It can also be beneficial for anyone who is taking heavy medication (chemotherapy, triple therapy, corticosteroids, etc.).

It then becomes a real manual medicine for bodies mistreated by the rhythms of modern society.

The therapist makes a complete assessment and provides care based on palpation, questioning, listening and observation of his patient. The result is an adapted, unique and personalized treatment. The focus is more on the person than on the disease. We try to understand his universe, his desires, his dislikes, his fears, his wishes, his projects. We look for the source of the problems and we try to restore the source of Life. This is the path I have been following for 40 years and I intend to keep on going this way!

Another aspect to this is the journey of the Way of the Heart. The care then becomes a wonderful opportunity to exercise compassion and a sense of service. By learning about the other we discover ourselves, and it is by going deep within ourselves that the other appears. It is in this permanent back and forth that the practitioner finds joy in his work. Thus, Shiatsu becomes a therapeutic art where the ultimate goal is not limited to the end of symptoms but to the experience of non-separation.

As they say in Japanese: *I shin den shin* ("From my heart to your heart").

And Ivan Bel's book also clearly emphasizes this aspect of things.

Indeed, although the therapist knows the great points, masters of the Breaths of the Body, he is above all immersed in a moment of immanence where the "being-bodies" are one and the same entity. The heart opens, touched by the suffering of the other, accepting being overlapped by it. The "other" disappears and the suffering with it.

This is the art of "Healing in Oneself". It is within this unity that secrets are told and read, and that a deep one-to-one relationship is woven. The sincere practitioner then makes the complete experience of the human "sometimes climbing higher than the eagle and sometimes crawling lower than the earthworm".

The balance he wants to transmit, he finds it in his loins; the peace of heart that he seeks to share, he discovers its harmonious melody in his chest; the equanimity he shares, he draws its source in his morning meditations.

The practitioner knows that the most valuable teaching is housed in his heart, and through his own, he invariably seeks the connection with his patient's inner physician. Then the healing force, within this "non-separation", achieves the experience of Oneness and can work deeply and often work miracles.

Strong in these virtues, the therapist becomes a companion on the way, a friend in the caring, a messenger between Heaven and Earth.

He knows that he is greater than himself and that great energies are at work when he "lets himself be found".

We then speak of the Way (Dō) and it is perhaps there that lies the secret of Shiatsu that makes the body vibrate and the heart sing. The practitioner then knows that he is not the master of his work, but that it is the Way that works in him. He does not act, he "is acted" by the force and presence of the breath-*Ki*.

This breath that runs through him is the same that blows the wind, the same that makes the Earth revolve around the Sun and holds the world together. The body is a small universe, and the universe is a large body.

The old Chinese and Japanese masters always wanted to account for this, and the poet Tagore sang it in his *Song Offerings*: "The same river of life that runs through my veins night and day, runs around the world and dances in rhythmic pulsations".[3]

This book by Ivan Bel will educate the student on the Way, awaken the practitioner on his path so that he exercises in all conscience the magnificent work of the Shiatsu therapist.

May this book guide you on this Path and connect you to the Spirit of Shiatsu as well as to the luminous forces of Life.

Thank you, Ivan, for opening the path of tradition and knowledge; each chapter is a step towards achieving Oneness with oneself, others and with the world.

Knowledge, Peace and Joy will ensue.

Master Ueshiba, founder of Aikidō (1883–1969), reminds us of this with these words: "The way of budo is to make the heart of the Universe one's own heart."[4]

Bernard Bouheret
Physiotherapist DE[5]
Shiatsu practitioner and teacher graduated from Hakko School (Japan)
Founding Director of the EST (Ecole De Shiatsu Thérapeutique)[6]
President of the Francophone Union of Therapeutic
Shiatsu Practitioners (UFPST)

Foreword

by Bill Palmer

S hiatsu has generated more different styles than almost any other therapy. In 1994, I was a plenary speaker at the International Shiatsu Conference in Melbourne alongside Ryokyu Endo, originator of Tao Shiatsu, and Sonia Moriceau, originator of Healing Shiatsu. The theme of the conference was to explore the evolution of Shiatsu. At the last moment, the Namikoshi family turned up in two limos. They took first place on the stage at the initial meeting and passionately denied the validity of the conference, saying that their Shiatsu was the only legitimate form.

If they had been the first to coin the word Shiatsu, I would have understood their position, but as Ivan Bel points out, Fukanaga Kazuma first used it to describe the therapeutic use of finger-based bodywork. However, the Namikoshis were the first to popularize it and get it officially recognized. I could feel their alarm at how the system they had developed was evolving out of their control. Talking to Ryokyu Endo about why he called his style Tao Shiatsu rather than just Shiatsu, he said that, in Japan, you could only become a master in your own right if you did something different to your Sensei. Japan's hierarchical culture did not allow many people to innovate and evolve *one* system. This may explain why, in its home country, there is a multitude of different forms of Shiatsu, many of which are essentially the same but with a small twist to differentiate them from their parent form.

Sonia Moriceau was not constrained by cultural hierarchy, but she felt that what she was teaching was essentially different to the Ohashiatsu that she had studied. She stressed the personal and spiritual development of the practitioner instead of the technical learning that Wataru Ohashi had emphasised at the time.

Another reason for the proliferation may be that, at its core, Shiatsu is so simple that teachers feel they need to add some bells and whistles to validate it as a serious subject to study. Whatever the reason, the many forms of Shiatsu have diluted its popular appeal. There is internal competition within the Shiatsu world, which gives mixed messages to the wider world. Rather than just expressing the simple fact that Shiatsu is a profound and wonderful therapy, different styles emphasize their differences and, in doing so, obscure the essence of this therapy.

Ivan Bel's book aims to connect all these forms to a shared stem. He defines the basic principles underlying almost all styles of Shiatsu and brings a refreshing sense of clarity and common ground to the confusion of many voices. Because his background was also in martial arts, he introduces valuable aspects of training that are not often included in Western Shiatsu schools. For instance, the practice of *misogi* is common in martial arts but almost unheard of in Shiatsu. *Misogi* is a training in endurance and, in Japan, usually involves staying in painful positions for a long time or repeating strenuous movements endlessly. The point is to learn to endure the agony and remain relaxed and centred through the pain. In Shiatsu, this develops the capacity to accompany clients through difficult therapeutic journeys without trying to rescue them. This illustrates another merit of this book: it reconnects Shiatsu to its roots in Japanese culture, which strengthens several capacities that are often overlooked in Western therapeutic training.

Lastly, this book embodies its author's personality. I see Ivan as a bright sword, cutting through confusion. The book essentially says to us: "Stop trying to be different! Stop over-thinking things! Remember the essential roots! Come together rather than continually dividing!" I agree that this is what the Shiatsu world needs: however different our styles may be, they are leaves on a tree with a common trunk and deep roots.

Bill Palmer M.Sc. ADPT FwSS
Co-Founder of the Shiatsu Society UK and Originator of Movement Shiatsu

Foreword

by Chris McAlister

Two friends and I had spent four months on the Indian sub-continent when, unexpectedly, the way opened over the daunting Himalayas into Tibet. The route was arduous, half built, the transportation at times non-existent, the scenery breathtaking in a literal sense.

On arrival, hungry mouths needed feeding. There were two or perhaps three problems standing in our way. First, an eatery had to be located and this was no easy task in a town completely unfitted to receiving travellers. Once located, the other problems presented themselves. The locals spoke no English, having never seen foreigners before. Equally and opposite, we spoke neither Chinese nor Tibetan. This initial problem was compounded by another, far more visceral obstacle.

After four months in India and Nepal, it had become second nature to us to imitate eating by holding our left hand out as a plate and miming picking up food with our (clean) right hand and delivering the food to our mouths. This method had earned us sustenance in wild, weird and wonderful surroundings. Here, suddenly, it was of no use whatsoever. We received blank looks and utterly confused body messaging in return.

What we gradually realized was that a whole other mimicry was required. One needed to cup the left hand into the shape of a bowl and, extending the long and index fingers of our right hands, imitate the action of lifting food with chopsticks from the bowl to our open, waiting mouths – from that moment on we never went hungry for very long.

The visceral, almost devastating impact was of having entered an alien world, one with completely different social rites and customs. What is the significance of this little story? It is that the language of the Indian subcontinent is wholly different to that pertaining to the broad stretch of land that starts with the Himalayas in the west of Tibet and extends all the way to the eastern coast of Japan. Naturally, there are considerable differences between these cultures, but the idea of eating rice or in fact almost any food with your fingers is completely foreign and quite distasteful to those residing there. Chopsticks represent the universal symbol for food, and mastering the art of eating with them will still gain you a basic level of respect in any of the countries and cultures you will meet between those two physical boundaries.

And what might be the relevance to our current situation? The book you are holding in your hands is the work of a man who has encountered similar situations, negotiated them successfully and entered worlds otherwise closed off to Western bodies and minds. The contents of this book have been earned with spirit, with will, with intention and with curiosity, but also with the blood, sweat and tears required to enter closed spaces and communicate with minds not always ready to share their knowledge at the mere drop of a hat.

What we have here is a very serious survey of the history of Shiatsu, meshed into a comprehensive presentation of its vigorous breadth and ancient depth.

The book is structured in accordance with the arcane symbology of earth, human and heaven, providing us with a simple method of entering into its contents wherever our interest might lie for the moment at hand.

Technique is dealt with in a detail never seen before – not from one approach but from several. Options and variations are presented with a fair and unbiased eye. Shiatsu is given room to breathe, to walk freely, to spread its wings and fly, and then return soundly to earth.

The book is lightened with tasteful illustrations depicting posture, grip, position and poise. Chinese characters are liberally but carefully employed to swiftly highlight concepts that are also explained at length in the well-written text.

A beginner, or one without prior knowledge of Shiatsu, might find elucidation in any of the chapters dealing with history, philosophy or basic technique. Students of Shiatsu will find not only detailed explanations of techniques they are already familiar with, but also alternatives not presented in the particular "style" or school they are currently engaged with. Practitioners will be reminded that their own story of Shiatsu is not and never can be complete – Shiatsu is always deeper, broader, more inclusive and more elusive than we can ever imagine.

What we have here is a gift to our still fledgling healing art form, a manual for the genuinely curious and a showcase to interest even the relatively uninterested. We are given this document, this living proof of the vitality of our method, with all its variation, its nuance and its ultimate indefinability: Shiatsu – a vital young branch on a venerable, ancient tree.

Chris McAlister
President of the European Shiatsu Federation
Practitioner and instructor of Shiatsu, acupuncture, Taiji and Qìgōng
Author of Touching the Invisible: Exploring the Way of Shiatsu and The Poetry of Touch: Alchemy, Transformation and Oriental Medicine

"Fate leads the one who accepts it and
drags the one who refuses it."

Seneca

"What has been twisted will be straightened."

Dao De Jing, Laozi

"Techniques imprison, principles liberate."

Léo Tamaki Sensei[1]

Acknowledgments

Writing a first book is a long-term adventure. This would not have been possible without the patience of my children and the constant love of my partner, friend and wife, Aurélie. The same goes for my parents who have shown unwavering support and love throughout my life. Without this force of unconditional love, I would not be where I am today.

In the world of Shiatsu, I would especially like to thank the regular support of Bernard Bouheret, a great man of French therapeutic Shiatsu and founder of the UFPST,[1] the Francophone Union of Therapeutic Shiatsu Practitioners, who from our first meeting believed in my abilities. I owe him a lot and not only for his corrections and encouragements to write this book.

I would also like to thank Frans Copers, pioneer of Shiatsu in Belgium and former president of the European Shiatsu Federation (ESF), who, from the height of his 40 years of experience, was also a source of unfailing friendship. In particular, he imparted to me the seven laws of natural health that form the third part of this book.

I also thank Hiroshi and Kikuno Iwaoka, both myo-energetic Shiatsu teachers in Paris, who helped me translate the Japanese terms and concepts. Thank you for the warmth of your friendship.

Finally, I would like to take this opportunity to thank all the masters I have met, who have all contributed to building my practice of Shiatsu. I want to acknowledge them here in order of meeting:

François Dufour (France), Françoise Bataillon (France), Lucy de Mooy (Holland), Yuichi Kawada (Belgium), Shigeru Onoda (Spain), Wataharu Ohashi (USA), Thierry Riesser (France), Akimoto Kobayashi (Japan), Kazuo Watanabe (Japan), Jean-Marc Weill (France), Raphael

Piotto (Belgium), Yasuhiro Irie (Japan), Stéphane Vien (Canada), Tzvika Calisar (Israel), Diego Sanchez (Uruguay) and Bill Palmer (UK). It is thanks to all these people that I am able to have such a broad vision of the universe of Shiatsu.

Preface

One always wonders how a book is born in the writer's mind. For my part, it was a situation and an observation that pushed me to it. One day when I was teaching Shiatsu, I was surprised that my advanced students had not yet understood what the essence of the technique is and all the inherent principles. "Come on," I exclaimed, "you still haven't understood the basic principles of our technique?" When I got home in the evening, I thought that these students were not to blame, since I had never formalized this part of the teaching for them. So, it was my fault. Then over time, I realized that none of the many Western teachers and Japanese masters I had met since my beginnings had ever explained it to me either. Admittedly, I had been told how to exert pressure and place my body, but that was about it. The rest was a set of more or less precise interpretations. I concluded that it was their fault.

However, even by exhaustively browsing my library and the many works on Shiatsu in it, I could not find any chapters on the fundamental principles that constitute this technique. There are plenty of books with theories and practical exercises, indeed, but almost nothing about the founding principles. I then immediately contacted my colleagues around the world to ask them the question and the answer was the same everywhere, apart from one author, one author whose book did address this subject but which is no longer in print.[1] Apart from that, there was nothing to be found, almost complete nothingness.

As with many things in Shiatsu, the oral tradition predominates. There are several good reasons for this. First, it is difficult to explain a kinaesthetic art. Words are only valid if the teacher can show and demonstrate them with his hands and body, essentially through

non-verbal language. It is obvious that this language cannot be reproduced in a book. This requires a living example. This is the reason why
technical books on Shiatsu show images that are useless without the
words of the master at the same time as his gesture in motion.

In short, a manual art is observed and felt. On top of that, in the
Asian spirit, we do not explain or we explain very little. We look and
we must "steal the technique with our eyes", a phrase that I have often
heard from the mouths of masters of martial arts and Shiatsu. To
put it another way, there is no pedagogy in Asia. Things are repeated
tirelessly until the mind lets go and the very depths of the body, the
muscles, tendons and even cells, at last understand. This method has
its good sides, but it does not help to teach accurately. The Western
mind possesses a force that pushes it to explain and analyse to teach
better. Do not believe that one system is better than the other. Asia and
the West do not oppose each other in this approach, but complement
each other, like Yin/Yang, in a permanent back and forth movement
between their two systems of thought and vision of the world.

By asking the question about the founding principles, I elicited
many reactions among Western teachers, each of them commenting
and contributing to my research. I have collected the opinions of
many great teachers from around the world – many I did not know
before beginning this long work – and for three years I made a difficult (and therefore imperfect) selection between what is part of
the essential principle and what appears secondary. This is how the
structure of this book was born little by little, to fill in the missing
parts of our understanding of Shiatsu, because as Laozi says in the
Dao De Jing: "What has been twisted, will be straightened out."

It must be understood that the practice of Shiatsu would be
ineffective without the very principles and concepts on which it is
based, which systematically combine the physical, the energetic and
the spiritual in a particularly harmonious and complete way.

With a lot of research, especially on the history of Shiatsu, I was
able to discover that very few principles were formalized during the
institutionalization of Shiatsu in Japan. After their defeat in the Second World War, Japan was under American influence to rationalize
and define all its sectors of activity, especially in the worlds of martial
arts and health. There used to be hundreds of manual techniques
that coexisted naturally. With the modern administration imposed

by the Americans, the Department of Health and Human Services had to put all this in order and required that, to be recognized, each discipline now had to define how it was unique and distinct from the others. In the world of manual therapies, the inability to do this meant returning to the familiar ground of Anma massage, whose studies and practice had been supervised for a long time. Dr Fujii oversaw the "Shiatsu" file, with an eight-year deadline to describe the specificity of this art and demonstrate its founding principles. He gathered around him a whole group of researchers, including doctors and Shiatsu teachers such as Tokujiro Namikoshi and his most brilliant young teacher of the time, Shizuto Masunaga. Without going into the various stages through which this research group passed, the final conclusions were as follows:

1. The paternity of the term "Shiatsu" goes to Tenpeki Tamai, author of the book *Shiatsu Therapy*.[2]
2. Shiatsu is performed by pressing with fingers, and especially thumbs, without the use of any tools.
3. The technical principles are fixed pressure, perpendicular pressure and continuous pressure.
4. The diagnosis is made at the same time as the pressure.

Thus, thanks to the definition of these few points, Shiatsu became an official branch of Japanese medicine and had its own state license from 1964. While Namikoshi was pleased with the situation, Masunaga thought it was only the beginning of defining the principles of Shiatsu. He had to go further. He devoted his life and all his efforts to the search for a broader philosophical and technical framework. In this research he was largely influenced by Zen, *Kanpō* medicine, Anpuku[3] and the work of various medical college professors. From there, the principles evolved and multiplied. Just one example: diagnosis. The *Shō* diagnosis was taken from *Kanpō* medicine and is divided into four stages: *monshin*, *bōshin*, *bunshin* and *setsushin*, the latter term often being contracted as *sesshin*. This method is now widely accepted in Shiatsu schools around the world as an integral part of the studies. Since the propagation of Shiatsu across the continents, it has been enriched with all the principles introduced by Masunaga. It is in this very broad spirit that I have listed the principles of Shiatsu in this book.

But why be interested in the principles of a therapeutic manual art? Because the technique is only a tool and tools can be used in an infinite number of ways. But technique tends to imprison those who only know that. On the other hand, the principles are few and mastery of them makes it possible to transcend the technique. Whether in martial arts or the arts in general (dance, singing, calligraphy, floral art, etc.), everything that comes to us from Asia is based on founding principles. They underlie the technique, like foundations that support an entire building. At a more advanced level, as we will see in the third part of this book, it is also philosophical and ethical principles that guide individual behaviour in practice. I have also added the energetic principles because Shiatsu is an art that uses the Qì as in Chinese tradition, Yin/Yang and many other theories. In this part I wanted to be as simple and practical as possible, without going into the many theories found in countless books.

When the principles are learned, integrated and become the very breath of the practitioner, he is then freed from the technique and can pull out all the stops. Let us make no mistake. Technique makes it possible to educate and work in a reassuring environment built in such a way that there is no risk for the student or practitioner.

But sticking to the technique does not allow you to discover the treasures that are hidden in Shiatsu. You must wear out your cloths and fingers many times to make the Shiatsu diamond shine. And for that, there are principles. One could argue they stem from a certain consistency that seems outdated, pedantic or overly formal that Westerners do not appreciate. And yet! Even a superficial examination of these principles shows that they are the only way to avoid deceptive appearances. Principles are guides that liberate, not shackles that enclose. They help to build and go beyond the technique, making the practitioner free and flexible, allowing him to adapt to any situation without ever judging or leaving his role, or modifying his art and diminishing his abilities. Quite the contrary.

I hope that this book opens the Shiatsu Way (*Shiatsu Dō*) to the greatest number of practitioners and brings them the necessary freedom for their practice.

Ivan Bel
Soulignac, January 2021

Vocabulary Warning

Although Shiatsu is a Japanese art, it is based on *Kanpō* medicine, literally "Chinese medicine". Therapeutic Shiatsu, as it is taught in the West, is therefore largely based on Chinese terminology. The mixing of Japanese and Chinese terms in a book does not make it easier for students or readers to understand.

That is why, in the following pages, I specify as often as possible the linguistic origin of the word. You will also find at the end of the book two glossaries, one with Japanese terms and the other with Chinese terms.

Regarding Chinese, the translation system chosen is pinyin, the system that has been in use since 1979.

The terms of Chinese medicine translated into English respect the usual nomenclature by starting with a capital letter, to distinguish them from the same notions in Western medicine. For example, the organ of the Spleen is not the spleen in the Western medical sense, and Blood in its Chinese sense covers many aspects unknown to blood in Western medicine.

Finally, regarding the term that refers to energy, I will use the term *Ki* (Japanese) or *Qì* (Chinese) depending on the context. So you will find both terminologies; please do not be offended.

Note that for ease of reading, "he"/"him"/"his", and also "Man" are used throughout most of this book. This should be taken to be inclusive of all genders and is not intended to suggest that all practitioners of Shiatsu and their clients are male.

Definition of Shiatsu

It is always good to be reminded of what Shiatsu is in order to define a framework. This technique has evolved so much in the last 20 years that often Japanese people who teach outside Japan are amazed at what has become of this art.

Above all, Shiatsu is a manual technique and a therapeutic art born in Japan. The term "Shiatsu" was first used by Fukanaga Kazuma (福永数間) who published *Chikara Ōyō Ryōhō Shiatsu-Hō* (力応用療法指圧法) (*Force Applied Therapy Finger Pressure Method*) in 1928, but this book has since been lost. He republished a second book under the pen name Tenpeki Tamai, *Shiatsu-Hō* (指圧法) (*Shiatsutherapy*, 1939). He is now officially identified as the founding father of Shiatsu. In this second book, he explains that the book is the fruit of 20 years of experience. This is why the birth year of Shiatsu is considered (until proven otherwise) to be 1919. Shiatsu was popularized in the 1940s by Tokujiro Namikoshi. During the 1950s, the Ministry of Health asked practitioners to make themselves known and to distinguish themselves from Anma massage, the oldest form of medical massage in Japan. This work of definition took several years, at the end of which Shiatsu was defined in 1955 by "the law on practitioners of Anma, Massage and Shiatsu, practitioners of Acupuncture and practitioners of Moxibustion". In 1957, the Ministry of Welfare (now the Ministry of Health, Labour and Welfare) published the book *Theory and Practice of Shiatsu*,[1] in which it is defined as follows:

> The Shiatsu technique refers to the use of fingers and palms to apply
> pressure to particular sections on the surface of the body in order to

correct imbalances in the body, and to maintain and improve health. It is also a method that contributes to the healing of specific diseases. In 1964, Shiatsu was recognized as a technique in its own right.

The Shiatsu therapist diploma gives access to official recognition in Japan, but not yet in the rest of the world. However, never has a manual technique met with such a large audience from the public. It only takes one session to immediately feel the beneficial effects. However, this is far from what we generally imagine a massage to be. There is no friction, no mixing, no flare-ups, nor any oil, since the recipient remains dressed. The fingers, mainly the thumbs, come to press on specific points or areas of the body. Relaxation on the one hand, and the feeling of re-energization on the other hand, make this technique a real art of caring. Everything is affected in such a way that the surface and depth are stimulated, that the musculoskeletal system as well as the organs are relaxed, that the mind and the body are harmonized and at peace with each other. The benefits of this technique are so numerous that it would take many books to describe them.

But what makes this technique? What are its mechanical, conceptual, philosophical principles? That is the purpose of this book which, I hope, will speak to the heart of experienced practitioners as well as neophytes.

Happy reading.

Earth

Basic Technical Principles

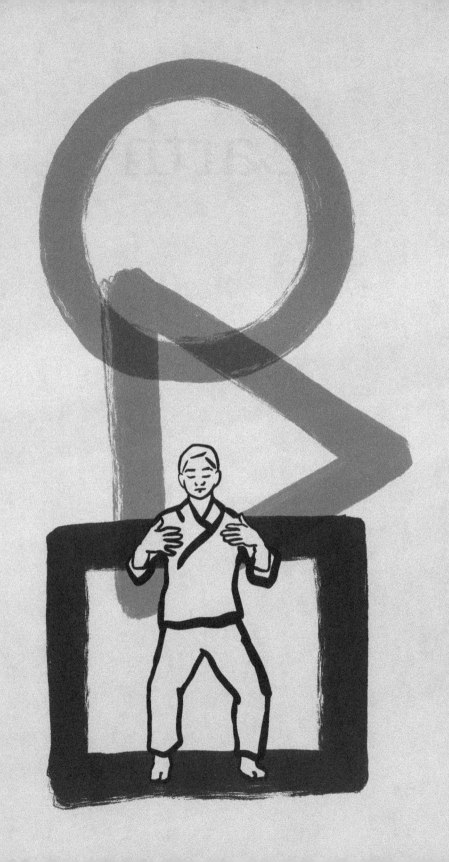

Explanation of the Basic Technical Principles of Shiatsu

A ll martial arts practitioners around the world must know their technical curriculum like the back of their hand; this allows them to make movements that are both aesthetic and powerful. But beyond appearances, each practitioner also knows and understands the basic principles behind their technique. These principles will guide them in the performance of their technique and serve as a safeguard so as not to stray from the path traced by their elders or lose sight of the heart of their art.

Thus, if we take the example of Karate, the shortest path between the fist and a target is a straight line. As a result, the attack movements of Karate are very direct with the basic principle of a straight-line attack. In contrast, Aikidō prefers the associated principles of *irimi* and *tenkan* (i.e., enter and pivot, often mistranslated as "dodge"), favouring movements in circles and spirals. The basic principles of the technique are therefore circular entry and displacement. Thus, each martial art offers a series of principles, guides and guidelines to propose a framework for the practice of the technique. In each martial discipline, we also see – just as in Shiatsu – that many branches, families and styles have developed from the unique teaching of a founder. This is usually a good sign because it proves the interest of the public and the vitality of the discipline. But even with many different branches of the same martial art, all practitioners will agree on the same basic technical principles, and sometimes on more philosophical principles. It is the very image of the tree with its many branches and a single common trunk to carry them all. It is at the trunk level that all branches can communicate, meet and exchange with each other. Defining the trunk is therefore crucial.

If Shiatsu has many points in common with Asian martial arts, one difference is that the great founders, Tenpeki Tamai, Tokujiro Namikoshi, Shizuto Masunaga, Tadashi Izawa, Yutaka Sakakibara, Ryuho Okuyama and Katsusuke Serizawa (to name only the best known), did not see fit to leave in black and white for the following generations the founding – and therefore unifying – principles that define what the Shiatsu technique is. And this is a great pity for the cohesion of this manual therapeutic art across continents and currents.

Let us then ask ourselves the question: what is a technical principle?

A principle is a mechanical, energetic, philosophical or spiritual notion that underlies and allows the correct realization of the technique and spirit of the technique.

The first reaction of some of my colleagues when I began writing this book was to say that energy is the first principle. From the point of view of technique this is a mistake, because the Shiatsu technique comes to rely on energy, which is not a principle but an immaterial phenomenon, omnipresent, unconditioned and external to the technique. Moreover, energy pre-exists from all eternity before the creation of any technique. The technique is at the service of energy, and not the other way around, because energy does not allow the physical realization of the Shiatsu technique. Energy supports the technique. Furthermore, there are many techniques that seek to mobilize energy, such as Seiki, Reiki, Qìgōng, Tàijíquán, Pranayama, etc. It is therefore important to understand that this first part consists in defining what makes it possible to achieve a correct technique, which, *ultimately*, can meet the energy. Finally, in the official texts of the Japanese Ministry of Health, the definition of Shiatsu never speaks of energy but of imbalances. However, all people who use Shiatsu as a daily work tool know that the notion of imbalance includes a vast field: mechanical, psychological, physiological and energetic.

All these areas are fully covered by the art of Shiatsu.

For the sake of simplification, I have chosen not to address the theories underlying the art of Shiatsu because they are those of traditional Oriental medicine (whether Chinese, Korean, Vietnamese or Japanese). There are many excellent books on this subject, and I refer the reader to authors such as Giovanni Maciocia, who is a leader in the field.

So, let's start with the basic principles that are all inseparable from the correct realization of the Shiatsu technique.

1

Perpendicular and Continuous Pressure

The world of Shiatsu represents a great diversity of practices, styles and schools. Just think of the styles of Namikoshi Shiatsu, Iokai Shiatsu, Zen Shiatsu, Kuretake Shiatsu, Kōhō Shiatsu, Yoseidō Shiatsu, Aze Shiatsu, Ohashiatsu, Yin Shiatsu, Shosei Shiatsu, Non-indō Shiatsu, Sei Shiatsu, Ryōhō Shiatsu and many others, and one immediately gets a glimpse of the great variety and richness of this art. This diversity shows the great vigour of Shiatsu throughout the world. All these styles work on ways of doing things and approaches that can be quite different from each other. But on the other hand, all practitioners of all styles agree at least on a first basic principle: perpendicular pressure.

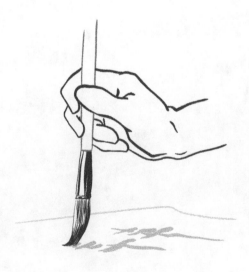

Indeed, this perpendicular pressure is the very heart of the way to approach the pressure points (ツボ *tsubo* in Japanese) of all meridians. By extension, this way of doing things is practised even outside of *tsubos* and has become the trademark of Shiatsu. Without this perpendicular pressure, you are *de facto* out of Shiatsu. For example, approaching tissues with fingers at an angle and sliding is the field of massage therapy, especially for working on fascia,[1] which is quite exciting but has nothing to do with our discipline.

Finding perpendicularity

To be done correctly, several mechanical factors need to be established for this type of pressure. The first is awareness of what perpendicularity is in relation to the area to be pressed. It seems enough to go from top to bottom to be sure about being perpendicular to the ground. But it's not as simple as it seems at first glance, because the human body is not a flat sheet of paper. It has many valleys and mountains, hills and hollows, varied and sometimes complicated topography. In short, it is three-dimensional. Therefore, it is necessary to read the body in sections and mentally make a kind of tube of each section, except for the head which is represented as a sphere. The pressure must always be applied towards the centre line of each tube or a central point for the cranial sphere. For example, the thigh, the pressure perpendicular to the floor will be on the top line of the thigh. But on the side, you will have to tilt your fingers a quarter, half or three-quarters to aim each time towards the centre line of the thigh. Respect this principle of perpendicularity to the centre and you will be using the pressure that is specific to Shiatsu.

To show perpendicularity to beginners, just use a tool of great technological precision and resulting from many hours of intensive research: the plastic water bottle! Place it on the body of a student lying on his stomach and move it over the hollows and bumps of the body while maintaining contact between the bottom of the bottle and the surface of the skin. The bottle tilts in one direction or another, which makes it possible to immediately apprehend visually the correct inclination of the fingers according to the topography. This method always gives the correct perpendicularity to any anatomical area of the human body. Thus, thanks to this very simple and very visual example, the student learns not to press at the wrong angle.

Now that perpendicularity is well defined, let's understand how the pressure works. For the pressure to be good for both the practitioner and the recipient, it must meet several criteria.

First, the posture of the practitioner respects essentially two positions (*seiza* and the kneeling knight), but here is the exhaustive list:

- sitting in *seiza* (legs folded under the buttocks, Japanese style)
- sitting in *kiza* (same position as before, but the toes are planted in the ground)
- seated in *tate hiza* (one leg raised forward and seated on the back foot)
- sitting in *iai goshi* (like the previous position, but the toes of both feet are planted in the ground)
- seated in *ryōhiza tachi* (upright on the knees, toes turned to the floor)
- half standing in *katahiza tachi* (semi-raised position called lunge position or kneeling knight).

These six positions meet specific needs that you will discover in the next chapter on body postures.

Pressure without force

Once the posture is correct, it is essential to check that the practitioner does not use muscle strength in the fingers, wrists, elbows and shoulders. The reason for the absence of voluntary force is dictated by the wide variety of anatomical realities of the human body. The tissues are thick, thin, sometimes there are bones under the surface, at other times we do not feel them, or we touch organs, or these are hidden in depth. Faced with the diversity of situations and bodily reactions that the fingers will encounter, it is not possible to make a technical catalogue of the different pressures to be carried out in each case. To achieve this, the founders of Shiatsu chose not to put force in the arms, hands or shoulders, but to move the body back and forth in order to move the centre of gravity of the practitioner. As a fortunate consequence, the body always exerts the right pressure, regardless of where the fingers are placed, without risk of injury. The mistake of beginner students is usually to add pressure with their muscular strength, believing they are doing well, which quickly causes unpleasant sensations or even pain in the recipient. On the other hand, the strongest of them are wary of their weight or power and, as a result, hold back and block the movement of displacement of the centre of gravity. In this case, the recipient often feels half-heard, half-accepted, and therefore half-treated. He also risks paying half of the advertised rate... Shizuto Masunaga recalls in his books that the two actors (giver–receiver) support each other, lean on each other, while maintaining a perfect balance between them. It's a beautiful image to keep in mind.

Pressure without force, by moving the practitioner's body back and forth, makes it possible to touch all areas of the body without any risk. Better, it also allows anyone (no matter their shape or size) to practise Shiatsu with the same efficiency. Students could be taught that *"The law of least effort is always the best in Shiatsu. So, stop overdoing it!"* Just let the body go without adding any pressure other than your own weight, a weight that can be easily managed by movement. This pressure will stop automatically in contact at the first resistance presented by the tissues, since there is no force. Thus, the practitioner identifies the resistance every time, without exceeding it and risking triggering pain or a myotatic reaction.[2]

It is generally accepted that correct pressure, to start acting on the body, is between 15 and 25 kilos of pressure. In fact it depends completely on the style of Shiatsu you study on the one hand, and the anatomical reality you encounter on the other hand.

It is quite surprising to know that, historically, Tokujiro Namikoshi exerted rather light and slow pressures. Yet today the Namikoshi school is known for its tonicity and speed of execution.

On the other hand, Masunaga applied very strong pressures, known to be painful. Today's Zen Shiatsu schools are rather gentle.

In some cases of big painful contracture, there is no point in putting a lot of pressure on the area to try to make the contraction go away. It will often be counterproductive, because the inflammatory or myotatic reaction will generate more pain and protection through over-contraction. In this case, it is better to have a light pressure. But when learning Shiatsu, the difficulty is to teach the student how to evaluate and feel on the one hand his natural pressure and, on the other hand, to know how to exert a precise pressure. To accurately measure the weight of a pressure, there is nothing better than a good old mechanical scale. The fact that it is mechanical is important, because with an electronic model it is impossible to follow the evolution of the pressure. The student then adopts one posture or another and applies pressure to the scale. He can control the pressure on the weighing dial and feel the weight in kilograms that he applies on the square centimetre of each thumb. I recommend developing pressure skills to be able to exercise this at will. Play regularly with the scales to feel what 5 kg of pressure represents, then 10, then 15, then 20, and so on until your maximum. Then challenge blindfolded practitioners or students to put exactly the right amount of weight without seeing the needle of the scales. You will develop an intimate knowledge of the pressure you choose to place, then come back to 15–25 kg in your treatment, depending on the size of your recipient. This is the average amount of pressure at which the practitioner encounters the human body's first resistance, without causing pain.

The three steps of pressure

The pressure on the body must also respond to three very specific steps that can be detailed as follows:

1. Placing your fingers without pressing: this is *coming into contact* with the surface.
2. Vertically pressing the surface to be treated: this is the *pressure*.
3. Gradually removing the fingers: this is the *release*.

These three steps are essential to the success of touch in Shiatsu. If you forget one of these steps, the recipient will immediately say that the gesture is unpleasant. It is also pedagogically interesting to test pressures omitting only step 1, then 2, then 3. In the first case, the pressure arrives directly and without introduction, which gives the sensation of being placed under a stapler. It is aggressive and generates a protective reaction on the part of the muscles. It is very difficult to let go with this type of touch. In the second case, the fingers arrive and then leave, without pressure. The feeling of not having been touched, listened to (manually speaking), is obvious. Basically, nothing happens. In the third case, removing the fingers abruptly at the end instead of gradually disengaging gives the unpleasant feeling that something is wrong, not being loved and not receiving appeasement. In any case, thanks to this simple exercise, the receiving student immediately becomes aware that the three steps in pressure support each other and that they are inseparable. If one is missing, the body immediately indicates that something is wrong. Of course, it is possible to spend more or less time on a particular stage in order to vary the pace of the Shiatsu, as we will see in Chapter 4.

Stable and continuous pressure

Perpendicular pressure in Shiatsu has two additional aspects. Perpendicularity occurs not only when placing the fingers but must be maintained throughout the duration of the pressure. This seems obvious, but it is not always the case when we watch beginners and even, alas, sometimes more advanced practitioners. When the pressure is engaged, there must be no more comings and goings, hesitations or tremors, otherwise the signal sent to the body is completely different from that of Shiatsu.

Furthermore, under no circumstances should the pressure deviate from its perpendicular axis and it should not slip. This is why stable pressure is the third most important aspect in Shiatsu pressure, a notion that was also set when the definition of Shiatsu was established.[3] We often see this error on the first points of the Bladder meridian at the top of the back. The student is in *katahiza tachi* (see the next chapter on positions) alongside the body of the receiver, ready to begin the Bladder meridian or the chain of the *Huá Tuó jiājǐ*[4] points (华佗交脊). But in doing so he will be in a bad position to touch the first three or four points that are located on the upper back, sloping towards the neck. And half the time the fingers slide and do not press the desired points correctly. This is typically an easy mistake to fix by positioning yourself above the head to do this part of the back, before moving alongside the back to do the rest. But more than the poor knowledge of placement around the body, slipping in pressure can also create a more or less disabling pain. Indeed, by slipping in pressure, it is possible to roll a nerve, tendon or muscle, which can hurt very much. I was unfortunately the victim of a bad technique of sliding counter-fibres on my rhomboids during a massage in Bali which immobilized my shoulder for four days. Only acupuncture (in the absence of Shiatsu on the island at that time) allowed me to regain movement and relieve pain. This experience confirmed for me the absolute necessity to respect the non-slipping of the fingers in pressure and to know anatomy correctly.

Three depths in pressure

Thanks to perpendicular, stable and continuous pressure, thanks to the three steps and the precise work on the amount of pressure, the practitioner can at last choose to enter more or less deeply into the tissues.

Let's be clear: this is possible as long as the progression is not stopped by tissue resistance. Some texts and schools describe seven levels of depth in a *tsubo*, but almost no one is able to feel or explain them. It's easier for everyone to divide the depth into three levels. This layout of depth in the pressure will make it possible to contact different tissues:

- On the surface: this is used to stimulate the skin, blood capillaries, nerves and surface sensors of the skin, but also the tiny communication meridians.[5]
- Mid-depth: to relax the subcutaneous layer and muscles and contact the meridians.
- In depth: to reach the organs, the deep nerves (especially those of the back or belly), the deep blood system, and the Extraordinary Vessels.

Depth also implies a choice in the treatment, because depending on the depth you may not come into contact with the same energy.

- On the surface: soothes, tranquilizes and stimulates the energy of the Yang meridians.

- Halfway: with half-pressure, stimulates the energy of the Blood.
- Deep: with complete pressure, stimulates the energy of the Yin meridians.

With these few remarks, we better understand the importance of mastering the basics of perpendicular pressure, because this directly influences the type of treatment we want to accomplish. We can therefore play with a whole range of pressures, provided we understand the benefits and the issues that arise from it.

By the way, this work of going from the surface to the depth, from external to internal, has a name in Chinese: it is the *Biǎo lǐ* (表裡) *relationship* (see the Glossary of Chinese terms at the end of the book).

Summary

1. Pressure must always be perpendicular to the anatomical centre of the pressure zone, must not slip, and must be stable.
2. The posture allows you to work without muscle force and to keep the correct pressure.
3. There are three inseparable stages within pressure: placing, pressure and release.
4. Perpendicular and forceless pressure allow you to adapt the depth for the treatment.

2

Postures of the Body and Fingers

As mentioned in the previous chapter, there are several postures in Shiatsu. Shiatsu is a Japanese discipline, and it is in the nature of the inhabitants of this country to codify the slightest gesture in all the arts and crafts they practise. This is also the case for their entire society, nothing escapes it. The goal is not to set the way of doing things in stone, but to teach the best. The quality of a technical gesture always depends on the use you make of your body: just think of an athlete, whether swimmer, javelin thrower or pole vaulter. The movements are worked on again and again and, to achieve this, a good study of posture is necessary. You can't imagine a sprinter positioning himself like a frog on the starting line, nor a javelinist with his back bent forward and his shoulders closed before launching his projectile. The posture is the basis on which the gesture is built and, consequently, the success of its movement. It is the same with Shiatsu, which is why the postures are both codified and very precise. As the practice of Shiatsu is traditionally done on the ground, it is important to master the sitting positions.

Seiza 正座

The first posture is *seiza* (正座). The person sits with both legs folded and the feet forming a seat for the buttocks. Purists, especially in *zazen*, will say that the left big toe must cover the right big toe, but without going that far, it is essential to check that the spine is in the centre between the two feet. *Seiza* literally means "correct, fair" and "sitting", which translates to "the correct way to sit". The practitioner, in the *seiza* position, with the knees far enough apart to get close to the recipient's body, is seated on a rock-steady base, which is an asset for stability. In this position, the pelvis is correctly positioned with the sacrum perpendicular to the ground. Thanks to the opening of the knees, the hips are also well open, which allows the belly (the *hara*) to come out freely forward and offer it all the space it deserves. The lumbar spine straightens automatically and, if you make the effort, the rest of the back aligns (dorsal and cervical). Better yet, this position encourages the pelvis to tilt forward, since nothing prevents it, which will create a back-and-forth movement in the natural axis of the pelvis. This mobility seems reduced, but it is a mistake to believe this. It is possible to train to move the pelvis in all directions (right, left, front, back, circular in one direction then in the other) while sitting in *seiza*, to keep a very useful freedom of movement and allowing you to get up effortlessly. Nothing is fixed in *seiza*, quite the contrary.

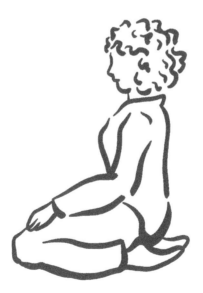

A good anchoring, the belly well cleared to offer deep breathing, a stable base, straight spine, the ability to move in all directions: *seiza* incorporates all the fundamental principles of a good posture, solid and flexible at the same time.

However, the *seiza* position has some drawbacks. First, it is not suitable for treating relatively large bodies, as is the case with obese people. In addition, many students (among Westerners) do not have the necessary suppleness of tendons and ankles, nor the sufficient muscle length of the quadriceps to tolerate this posture for long. It is certainly possible – and very healthy – to train and loosen up, but it takes several years to modify your body without too much effort.

Kiza 危座

This posture is the same as *seiza*, but for *kiza* (危座) the toes are turned against the ground, which allows a little more height. The other benefit is to gain mobility. Indeed, thanks to the tension in the soles of the feet, it is easier to give an impulse to move, while the knees can be raised and oriented easily. With the *kiza* posture, the practitioner gains mobility. Practitioners of Iaido or Aikido[1] are familiar with this position, as it helps them move easily on the ground with sometimes astonishing speed. And contrary to what one might think, it does not wear out the knees.

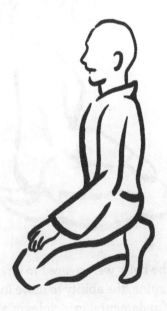

Chōki 長跪

The third position, *chōki* (長跪), consists of straightening up on the knees, while keeping the toes against the ground. Literally it means "long and kneeling", but it is also known as *ryōhiza tachi* (両膝立ち), in other words "standing on the knees". This is useful for treating larger bodies that require more height, when *kiza* does not allow it, such as the back of a person lying on a large abdomen. It is important to spread the knees to avoid imbalance. It is better to open them to the width of the hips to ensure two stable anchor points on the ground. This posture respects all the basic principles seen above. On the other hand, it is not comfortable for long and wears the knees because the kneecaps are directly on the ground. This posture can only be temporary during a treatment.

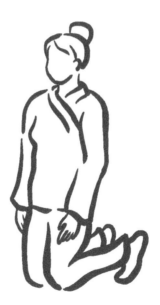

Tate hiza 立膝

This position is halfway between a sitting position and a more "raised" position. It comes from the depths of samurai culture because it allows sitting with a sword on the belt. *Tate hiza* (立膝) consists of sitting on one foot and placing the other leg forward, the knee raised to the sky. The rear foot is flat, with the top of the foot against the ground. As part of the art of the sword, this allows you to jump or get up quickly. In Shiatsu, this position is restful and allows you to vary with other positions to relieve the risen leg, allowing the blood to circulate. The only disadvantage in Shiatsu is that this position tends to push us a little too far from the body of the *jusha* 受者 ("receiver"), which forces us to bend our back to reach it. It can therefore only be a passing position, to stretch one leg after the other.

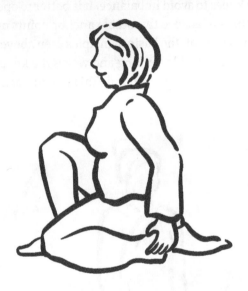

Iai goshi 居合腰

At first glance, *iai goshi* (居合腰) is very similar to *tate hiza*. The only difference is in the support: all the toes are turned against the ground. It doesn't sound like much, but this little detail really makes all the difference. First, with all ten toes under tension, it is easier to move along the recipient's body. In addition, unlike the previous position, it is possible to open the support leg further and get even closer to the *jusha*. From then on, the *shiatsushi* (the donor) regains the verticality of his backbone. In martial arts, using a katana, this position allows you to draw and move in the blink of an eye. We could say that this position is somehow more combative, more mobile than all other postures and not tiring for the legs.

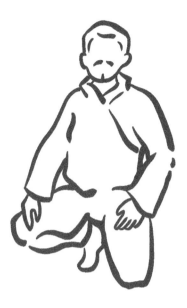

Hanza 半座

The last posture is *hanza* (半座), literally "half sitting", and therefore by extension "half standing". It is also known as *katahiza tachi* (片膝立ち) whose translation is "standing on one knee". In French, we say "lunge position" or "position of the kneeling knight". This is by far the most emblematic position of Shiatsu and it must absolutely be mastered. Just like when the knight is knighted, it is an act of humility by bending one knee forward and placing the other back and on the ground. The two legs form a 90-degree angle at the knees while the two feet are placed on two parallel lines to ensure good stability. If they are aligned on a single line, the practitioner finds himself in precarious balance, as if he was walking on a tightrope. To increase the ability to move, the toes of the back foot are planted in the ground. As with the other positions, the pelvis is wide open to let the belly pass to the front of the body. It is constantly oriented in the direction of the pressure zone, where the thumbs are, and in no other direction under penalty of creating a twist at the lumbar level.

This position is both pleasant and effective in terms of ability to move and exert pressure. In addition, it makes it possible to gain height and ensure perpendicular pressure on the part of the receiver most exposed to the sky (belly, back, flank or chest, depending on the position). Above all, it offers the ability to treat large areas without having to move too frequently or change direction quickly. However, it has several potential problems: fatigue of the lower back which will tend to arch, ditto for the upper back which will tend to bend, as well as potential pain in the pelvis at the joint level, especially in the inguinal region. In this case, the *shiatsushi* will seek to support his elbow on the thigh that is raised, thus reinforcing the defects in the posture without bringing lasting relief. Worse, by pressing his arm on the leg, the fingers will transmit its movements and vibrations. In these cases, the basic principles of the posture are compromised and will wear out the cartilages of the spine and joints and cause more fatigue, less breathing capacity in the belly, and less and less pleasure in practising Shiatsu. After a while this can mean students or practitioners abandon Shiatsu simply because of ignorance of postural principles. With a little will and awareness, all these problems can be solved by taking up one by one each principle of the posture. Despite this, this posture remains difficult for students who already have knee or back pains.

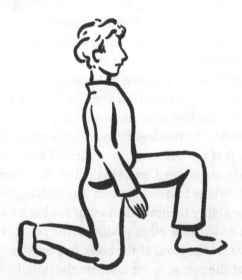

We advise people who have this kind of problem to work on a massage table when they cannot work directly on the ground. Moreover, we can note a clear evolution of tabletop work in the world of Shiatsu.

In Japan, many practitioners use a massage table. However, the standing posture is specific and requires lowering the table to half the height of the practitioner's thigh. Then, so as not to get tired in a standing position, it is beneficial to press both thighs against the edge of the table when working from the front. In some cases, the practitioner must get on the table to successfully execute certain movements, and especially to avoid lumbar torsion. It is highly recommended that the practitioner acquires a reinforced table to support the weight of two people. Working on the ground remains the reference, however, because this is how Shiatsu was created by its founder.

Stretching the spine

The spine is the central axis of the body, the trunk through which all our sensations pass thanks to the nervous system in our spinal cord. The spine's natural double curvature allows it to bend and stretch, in short to move. Ideally, the back should be as "straight" as possible, to not create a pinching of the nerves by the vertebrae. But straight does not mean rigid. During my student years, I believed for a long time that by keeping my back strictly straight I would never hurt myself. It was the opposite that happened because of the muscle contractions (tetany) I was inflicting on my back muscles. No, the ideal is to maintain movement in the column to avoid fatigue. The back-and-forth movement of the centre of gravity towards the body of the receiver is accompanied by a tilt of the pelvis. This rocking movement looks a bit like that of a rider who never remains frozen in a saddle, which could well compress all his vertebrae. Thanks to this rocking movement, the column waves back and forth with the pelvis going from retroversion to anteversion. Better yet, it constantly mobilizes the lumbar region and avoids pain in the area of the quadratus lumborum (the deepest back muscle). To become aware of this movement, it is interesting to grab both hips and feel the rocking of the pelvis in order to integrate it into your practice.

If the lower back moves, what about the upper back? The Canadian teacher Stéphane Vien teaches a very useful trick to avoid blockages at the top of the column. He encourages imagining the head as a balloon inflated with nitrogen, light and pulling upwards. For this he recommends making a "long neck" when the body goes forward, movement that is found in Tàijíquán. This consists of stretching the head upwards while tucking the chin in. Thus, we keep the cervical vertebrae in the axis of the spine. Then we release this slight tension in the return movement, at the same time as the pelvis goes backwards, to stretch the lumbar vertebrae. Thus, the spine is constantly mobilized and stretched following the back-and-forth of the practitioner's body.

I advise practitioners to not keep their eyes constantly on their fingers to avoid tension in the neck. Forgetting your fingers and looking ahead also means allowing yourself to feel with the whole body and therefore to increase your inner presence at the expense of the mind, as we'll see further on.

Movements of the pelvis

In the centre of Man is the large joint of the pelvis. It is called *koshi* (言霊), which encloses the *hara*, a notion that designates the belly but also much more than that. Indeed, in the Japanese mind it designates not only the centre of digestion, but also the energy centre, the centre of gravity, as well as the centre from which all movements spring. In the Far East, no art, no craft, no gesture is done without starting from the *hara*. The practitioner's job is to move his centre of gravity back and forth, a movement that is therefore initiated in the *hara*. This is possible thanks to the forward (anteversion) and backward (retroversion) tilt of the pelvis, for any of the postures we've just studied. This movement will make it possible to send weight forward and transmit it mechanically – via the arms – to the fingers to apply pressure. By tilting forward, the pelvis drives the spine and upper body, which adds further weight to the pressure. Be careful: the inclination of the upper body should always be the result of the inclination of the pelvis. Unfortunately, we often see the opposite because this movement is less tiring. It is not uncommon during workshops to see *shiatsushi* working by throwing the upper body forward to apply pressure. This is a profound ignorance of movement in Shiatsu. By using the upper body rather than the lower, the movement freezes at the diaphragm, blocks breathing, moves the shoulders up to the ears and does not exude the benevolent power found in a global movement that engages the whole body. In addition, in the long run, this technique tires the upper back and pain occurs after a few months because the posture in the movement is not respected.

It really is essential to engage the *hara* forward. From a mechanical point of view, we can say that the movement comes from the depths of the body, from the *seika tanden*, and exudes a quiet power that is both reassuring and effective. On the other hand, movement from the stomach cannot be as intrusive as movement from the upper back and shoulders because the latter requires the use of muscles, while the pelvis uses only the displacement of the centre of gravity, the displacement of the weight of the body. In this version of the movement, no muscular aggressiveness interferes and, possibly, hurts the recipient. On the contrary, this movement releases a deep and gentle pressure at the same time, which always stops on the tissue layer in tension, without ever doing any harm. From an energy point of view, the use of *hara* changes everything. With the rocking of the pelvis, the *shiatsushi* opens and offers his belly towards the patient. In other words, he gives his centre and opens himself to the other. The result is the feeling of being accepted, integrated, supported, recharged and loved. These words might make you smile, but you will see with years of practice that this notion is in fact an integral part of good-quality Shiatsu. This is why it is imperative to constantly use the back and forth of the pelvis as the basis of the Shiatsu technique.

Do not forget either that it is also the pelvis that comes back. This return movement makes it possible to disengage from the pressure. Do not raise your fingers or elbows or pull on the muscles in the middle of the back to remove pressure. This disengagement of the fingers from pressure comes from the pelvis withdrawing. Thanks to this, the return is smooth. Better yet, the fingers accompany the decompression of the tissues, which return to their place, and the recipient feels taken care of until the last moment, when the fingers disconnect. So, in any case, it is always the pelvis that is the main engine of Shiatsu.

Opening the shoulders

One common detrimental postural error is the forward closure of the shoulders. Students, especially those who use the upper body rather than the pelvis, will tend to stretch their arms to apply finger pressure, which will automatically close the shoulders forward. This could be amusing if the consequences were not serious. First, closing the shoulders requires contracting the top of the pectorals. Like any muscle contraction repeated too often, this will tend to create a permanent tension that will not go away. Second, closed shoulders impede good breathing in the chest, particularly by slowing down the passage of air in the bronchi. If you already know the Lung meridian, you know that you're closing the energetic circulation of its first two points. Given the importance of the respiratory function in physical and mental relaxation, it would be a shame to deprive oneself of it.

In addition, the contraction of the top of the rib cage will have an impact, admittedly moderate, on the cardiac region. But in the long run this will have deleterious effects. It is no coincidence that the most common pathologies among Shiatsu practitioners are heart disorders[2] (also joint problems in the knees and thumbs). It is therefore essential to regularly carry out exercises that open shoulders and breathing, not forgetting to check one's position during pressure. Certainly, the fact of joining the thumbs on a point tends to close the shoulders; it is then necessary to slightly relax the elbows and open them on the sides. The Aze Shiatsu school offers a trick which consists in moving the little fingers down the sides, whereas we tend to place them forward. One last solution, seen in Sei Shiatsu, is to let go in the pressure, to relax, even if it means letting the shoulders go up, to keep the chest wide open.

Finger positions

Even if we do sometimes use elbows, knees, feet or forearms, Shiatsu is mainly practised with the fingers and more precisely with the thumbs. Again, codified postures impose precise finger positioning. Besides, if you don't already know it, the word Shiatsu literally means "fingers" (指) and "press" (圧). There are several ways to place the thumbs depending on the different schools and styles, but for the basic study of Shiatsu it is highly recommended to place them side by side, or one on top of the other. This positioning of the thumbs makes it possible to create a triangulation between the two shoulders and a central point formed by both thumbs. Thus, the force released – by the back-and-forth movement of the practitioner's body – will focus on a very small area, again increasing the pressure capacity, without having to make any physical effort, while developing a very effective penetration angle (tip of the triangle).

The thumbs can be placed at two angles of approach:

- *Nigate gata* 苦手形: in this form, the tip of the thumb is stretched forward and presses on the tissues, which gives a piercing effect. Sometimes an action with the nail is added to punctuate a point or enter a small space, such as between the metatarsals of the foot.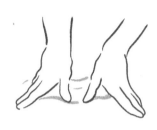

- *Amate gata* 甘手形: the other form places the last phalanx of the thumb flat, a more agreeable, softer pressure to receive since the pulp presses on the tissues. So that it does not get damaged by the folding of this joint, the *shiatsushi* seeks to align the bones from thumb to shoulder. This last point is essential to the realization of a technique without force, but especially without risk of thumb injury in the long run.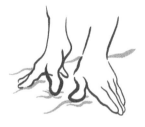

The pressure on the thumb is often strong. Without the effort of aligning the bones, the articulation of the first phalanx springs forward, while the articulation of the second phalanx goes backwards to be able to put the thumb flat. Instead of creating a single deviation of the thumb, there are now two, which means two weak points on small joints that are not made to bear such a weight load. To compensate for this, the great palmar muscle must tense up, which tires it and makes the whole hand lose strength, not to mention the risk of cartilage wear, tendinitis and elongation that would put a painful and sudden stop to your Shiatsu practice. Admit that would be a pity! It is therefore necessary to straighten the first joint of the thumb in towards the palm to get a straight thumb (with the exception of the last phalanx necessarily pressing on the body of the receiver). Once this is done, the radius bone is then aligned. The elbows should not be stretched but slightly relaxed in semi-extension (for the reasons just discussed). Also, be careful not to completely flex the elbows during pressure: this would remove all the force that you've released with the pelvis. Finally, the shoulders are low and open. In this way, any movement of the pelvis is immediately transmitted to the tip of the fingers, by the superposition of bones, without having to force. So you are then always more efficient without any great effort or risking penalizing yourself in the short or medium term.

Also remember to open all the fingers to distribute them on a large area, to stabilize the thumbs. Generally, the pressure is light on the fingers, and strong on the thumbs, which are the main actors of Shiatsu. However, schools sometimes change this rule to use a wider pressure and relieve the thumbs. This can be interesting when you want to work large muscles, as in the back: it is then better to apply pressure with the palm of your hand. In addition, by distributing the pressure on all the fingers we diffuse the pressure, the signals of the thumbs, placed on specific points, is eased, which means that we lose efficiency. Indeed, the recipient no longer knows whether to focus on the sensation of one finger or another. He cannot identify ten pressure points at the same time, the brain is not capable of it. It can only sense one or two pressure points, and rarely more. To conclude, as we are used to saying, *less is more*. By doing less, by being more precise, the transmission of the message and the efficiency of the treatment are increased. Therefore, it is better to put pressure on the thumbs, the other fingers being there to ensure stability.

As noted above, there are many positions for the thumbs, and even fingers. No matter which placement of the thumbs you have studied, the important thing is to respect ergonomic principles, namely: avoid creating breaking points at the level of the fingers, align the bones up to the shoulder, do not force muscularly. You'll thus ensure a sustainable practice of Shiatsu whilst respecting your own anatomical comfort.

Relationship between upper body and thumbs

As you will have understood, movement is constantly initiated by the pelvis and transmitted to the entire trunk, which leans forward. The movement is transmitted by the arms to the thumbs and allows the correct pressure, neither too strong nor too soft, thanks to the creation of an isosceles triangle formed by the chest and the two arms, the thumbs representing the penetrating tip. But there is a crucial point for the success of pressure: it is the centring of the hips in relation to the position of the thumbs. The thumbs must, to be effective, always be in front of the *hara* and more particularly the point which is three fingers below the navel. Admittedly, this movement can seem a little rigid and reminiscent of marionettes with their straight bodies and their stiff arms. But as we have seen before, nothing is stiff in the movement, so do not worry. On the other hand, a straight line between the centre of the *hara* and the thumbs is the most effective way to transmit the correct pressure.

What happens when the *hara* is no longer centred on the thumbs? First of all, we notice that the body twists to one side. Therefore, the breath can no longer go down into the belly. This is a shame because breathing well helps the practitioner relax, and allows them to put more weight into the application of pressure. Without breathing into the belly, the transmission of weight to the fingers isn't as effective, particularly because one arm will be farther away than the other from the pressure zone. But the most serious issue is undoubtedly the twist that is created at the lumbar vertebrae level. In the long run, this twist can cause a lot of damage to the intervertebral discs (lateral crushing, protrusion) and to the spinal nerves that come out on each side of the spine (from simple pinching to wearing out the nerve itself).

To preserve your body and the pleasure of practising Shiatsu in the long term, it is therefore imperative to constantly maintain the thumbs in front of the pelvis. The best exercise for students to work on this issue is working lines on the back in the kneeling knight position. The back being quite long, it is impossible to do all the applications of pressures with the pelvis in the same direction. It is therefore necessary to rotate it little by little, pressure by pressure, in order to keep it in its triangle with the thumbs. This movement of tracking the thumbs with the hips, called "sunflower", makes it possible to respect one's anatomy (especially, but not only, the lower back) and to distribute an equal pressure over the entire length of the back.

Summary

1. Shiatsu postures are codified and precise to not wear out the practitioner in the long run. But if it is anatomically impossible for you to respect them, then work on a table.
2. The correct posture allows the implementation of three principles: stability of the body, verticality of the back and opening of the belly.
3. There are six positions for practising Shiatsu: *seiza*, *kiza*, *ryōhiza tachi*, *tate hiza*, *iai goshi* and *kathizizachi*.
4. The mobility of the spine in movement prevents it wearing out and avoids pain.
5. The pelvis is the basis of the movement. It must always be located in front of the thumbs.
6. The correct posture increases the amount of pressure. So that the thumbs can support it in the long run, it is necessary to rectify their posture and align the bones from the fingers to the shoulders.

3

Stability

I magine that you are receiving a good Shiatsu. Suddenly, the fingers of the practitioner begin to tremble or to slip accidentally, or their whole body vibrates in an uncontrollable manner. For a receiver, there is nothing worse than feeling fingers shaking (when it was not planned). Predictability in movement, in repetition, in gestures and even in the ritual of a Shiatsu session is a highly reassuring factor for the person who comes to see you; especially if the receiver is physically (which is usually the case) or psychologically (quite common as well) weak. Never make sudden gestures or uncontrolled movements: the suspicion of a lack of professionalism and/or technical quality will immediately slip into the receiver's mind. This is why the principle of stability is one of the pillars on which Shiatsu is built.

In Shiatsu, stability is called *antei* (安定), which literally means "calm and determined". It concerns several aspects for the practitioner: musculoskeletal stability, psycho-emotional stability, and stability in presence. Make no mistake: these three aspects are intimately linked. Try giving a Shiatsu session after arriving late for your appointment. You were caught in traffic jams, you feel annoyed, you ran to your place of practice, you're thinking about not finishing too late to run errands or pick up the kids later... You can be sure that the recipient will feel all the disorders that agitate you, without you even needing to say a single word. This is why it is recommended to be well prepared before the first session of the day, to warm up and meditate so that the body is warm and the mind serene.

Physical stability

As soon as we feel the fingers vibrating, we can easily suspect that they are under too much pressure or that they are suffering the effects of physical fatigue. This is tantamount to saying that you're putting strength into your applications of pressure and that after a while the thumbs weaken, especially the joints of the phalanges and the great palmar muscle. Let's repeat it here: in Shiatsu you must not put strength into applications of pressure. If finger trembling is the result of an uncontrollable movement of the whole body, you are either poorly positioned in your posture, or leaning on your thigh in the so-called "lunge" posture, or completely exhausted.

In short, it's time to rest – take the necessary time – to recover deeply. Also take the opportunity to ask yourself what's wrong with your posture and eliminate flaws to find ease and comfort in practice. Calling your old teacher is also a good idea to discuss this with or possibly have your posture corrected.

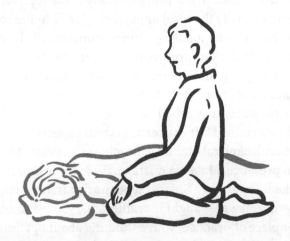

The stability of the thumbs, as we have seen, is greatly helped by the alignment of the arm bones. But the other fingers are not absent from the work. They must not be folded. On the contrary, the four other fingers must rest on the body of the receiver to stabilize the entire hand. With five points of support, one of which adds the pressure, logically you'll have better stability than on a single point of support and pressure. In addition, it will distribute the weight load of the practitioner and will strain the thumb less. Better still, it will allow you to discover new methods of applying pressure, to increase it with little effort, to play on wider areas, or to work with your little finger to stimulate your Heart meridian. Did you know that many practitioners complain of pain not in the thumb, but in the little finger? Yet this one is called in martial arts the "finger of strength". Indeed, it is easier to release a grip that uses the index and middle fingers than the ring and little fingers. But forgetting to use your little finger weakens it and thus weakens the Heart meridian, which in turn weakens the heart organ.

Having said that, the same problem of heart disorders can be found in practitioners of kinesiology, magnet therapy, and other forms of psycho-energetics, which would suggest that it is not only a mechanical question. We may think that too many emotional charges go through these practitioners, which over the years must weigh on their emotional system, or that practitioners do not do enough personal work on opening the Heart, including meditation. "Meditation washes the Heart of all its scoria," says Bernard Bouheret.[1] That is absolutely true. We will come back to this throughout this book. To conclude, we can say that the work of all the fingers is fundamental for the stability of pressure and the emotional health of the practitioner.

Of course, musculoskeletal stability is not possible without a minimum of work on oneself. Physical activity and sport maintain a healthy and strong musculoskeletal system. This will help you to trust in your abilities, your arms, your fingers. On days when you are tired, you will also be able to count on the resistance of the body. Stretching and mobility exercises help a lot as well. A flexible body has few tensions that may vibrate when there is fatigue. In addition, a regularly stretched body is easier to move and less likely to be injured by making a wrong move.

This physical stability also gives you the opportunity to focus on listening and feeling with your fingers in contact with the treated area, without being physically and mentally parasitized by an unwanted vibration. As a result, you can manage your pressure exactly according to the reactions of the body. You can also maintain pressure for as long as you wish, without experiencing short-term fatigue. But above all you give the receiver time and confidence to feel and work on himself, accepting tensions and emotions that disturb him to better surpass them. In other words, you are giving the receiver the necessary free space to do the therapeutic work at his own rhythm.

Psycho-emotional stability

Psycho-emotional stability goes far beyond the scope of this book, yet we must say a word about it. This inner balance between your mind and your emotions is essential to the quality of your Shiatsu. The more serene and carefree you are, the more you will be open to others, listening to your sensations. On the contrary, anxiety, worry and chaotic thoughts will destabilize your technique and can even weaken you, allowing an excess of untimely reflections. Therefore the job of the Shiatsu practitioner is also to ensure his mental balance, to continually learn to know himself better and to self-evaluate. It is always useful to ask yourself a few questions regularly:

- How do I feel?
- Am I happy today?
- Is my heart serene?
- Is my mind calm?
- If not, what are my resources and techniques to improve or calm down?

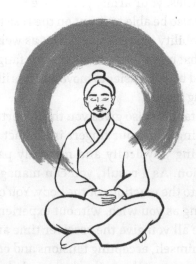

CALMLY SELF-EVALUATING TO GET TO KNOW ONESELF.

Over the course of your life as a practitioner, you will probably have to deal with patients who affect you more than others. This is especially the case when a person completely shares his feelings and his story; some stories we are not prepared for. This is also the case when a receiver discharges a large amount of energy that was blocked for a long time, or on the contrary, drains all your energy like a vacuum cleaner.

Emotional decompensations are not uncommon in this profession, and it is not always easy to face a person who curls up and cries a flood of tears, especially when you are starting out. To preserve oneself, to cleanse oneself too, it is recommended to take stock from time to time under the supervision of a more advanced practitioner, or to follow a brief psychotherapy intervention to get help on personal blockages.

Let's take an example: a woman tells you about her rape and is angry against all men. If you are a man, you may feel blamed and unconsciously responsible for her suffering. This mechanism is called a psychological breach, a situation that shifts you from your role as a therapist to that of an aggressor. Do not keep this disorder in yourself and get help as soon as the situation starts making your thoughts go in circles or deprive you of sleep. Furthermore, if many people come to rely on your expert fingers, you must accept to do the same, if only out of humility. It is dangerous to think that you are all-powerful and that care is only for others.

Inner presence stability

To improve psycho-emotional stability, meditation is one of the most valuable tools. If we stick to the perception of the human being according to Taoist philosophy, it is composed of a body, a mind (brain) and a higher consciousness that could be translated as "soul". By learning inner silence and physical stillness, meditation gradually opens a calm and deep inner space in which nothing disturbs you. This free space will expand and, over time, will put you in communication with your higher consciousness. To listen to what this awareness has to tell you, you must develop a great sense of listening and attention to yourself.

This work will be very beneficial to you in Shiatsu since this silent listening is essential to feel – and even "see" – with your hands what is happening in the other. This inner presence, this availability of body and mind, is immediately felt by any recipient. He will often tell you that the session was incredible, when technically you did not do much, or even almost nothing. But the greater your presence, the deeper the treatment. This depth is the mark of the great masters of Shiatsu.

Meditation will bring you many benefits. First of all, by spending time observing your breathing, you increase its quality and oxygenate your cells properly. Thanks to the lotus or *seiza* position (depending on which one you prefer), your posture, your verticality and therefore your perception as a human being will evolve towards greater physical and moral quality. Not only will your inner presence improve your ability to listen to others, but also to your own feelings. This detail is important in order to know if everything is fine, or if you are "tying yourself in knots". Moreover, a good meditation can undo muscle knots or blockages in the spine. This reminds me of an anecdote. I did Zen meditation for a long time, and I always tried to have a straight back, like an "i". When I started Kawada Sensei's class, he looked at me in *seiza* for a little while. Then he said to me: "This is not good. The spine must move with the breath, there must be movement in the immobility otherwise you will have back pain." And indeed, I inevitably suffered from back pain during meditation sessions. Since I move my spine with the movement of breathing, it has become a pleasure to stay "still".

Finally, the last point I want to talk about with meditation: developing the ability to be in the present moment will help you to not have a thousand thoughts interfering with the messages sent by your hands and the silent communication that is inevitably established between your Qì and that of the recipient. All this explains why most practitioners who accumulate an experience of more than 20 years declare that Shiatsu is a meditation in motion, a time without thought, totally in listening to what is at stake at that moment.

Thanks to these three stabilities, you are fully available for your Shiatsu and the person who is with you. The recipient will feel it deeply and will feel greatly supported and listened to, even if the session goes without a word. Of course, it is also good to let off steam sometimes. A good jog or the practice of martial arts helps to balance your psyche through physical activity and help to savour even more the return to inner calm. Remember: every Yin needs its Yang, and vice versa.

Summary

1. A lack of stability will affect the quality of your Shiatsu.
2. The stability of the whole body is achieved through posture. But that of the thumbs is provided by the support and use of other fingers, which must never be forgotten.
3. Stability also involves the maintenance of the mechanical body.
4. Stability is also psycho-emotional. You need to work on yourself as often as possible, ideally every day.
5. Meditation develops inner stability and increases greatly the ability to listen and pay attention. It "washes the heart" of all the imprints of the sessions.

4

Rhythms

There is a lot to say about rhythm when it comes to Shiatsu. Shiatsu is a therapeutic art[1] intrinsically linked to Far Eastern medicine in the broad sense. This itself is entirely related to the movements and rhythms of nature that ancient Taoists and Shintoists observed for millennia. It is therefore logical that Shiatsu is the very representation of these rhythms and translates them within its technique. This is also the reason why some schools teach sequences such as Fire, Metal, Earth, Wood and Water in the corresponding season, in order to put their students in tune with these energetic movements of nature.

However, each style of Shiatsu seems to have crystallized around a precise rhythm in pressure, to the point of making it their distinctive trademark. On the one hand, this specialization is interesting because it has made it possible to study thoroughly what a particular rhythm can do on the human body, in addition to the perpendicular pressure and its depth. Take for example Kōhō Shiatsu or Jigen Ryū Shiatsu, which have a very fast rhythm (of the order of a second) and a fairly strong pressure, while on the other hand Zen Shiatsu or Yin Shiatsu can spend a relatively long time on each point. On the other hand, these specializations stop us from appreciating all the rhythms of pressure and using them all. It's a bit like telling a mechanic to use only the size 12 spanner and not touch any other to repair an engine, or telling a musician to play only one note. Sounds disabling, doesn't it? This is indeed the case.

The different rhythms

Between the two extremes (very fast and very slow), there is a whole range of possibilities. They can be classified more or less as follows:

- **Less than 1 second**: these are precise strikes to perform a *kuatsu* (resuscitation technique) when a body weakens severely or just after trauma.
- **1 second**: very fast, this rhythm is used in Shiatsu of martial origin. It tones the body and the Yang. For this type of Shiatsu, it is better to already be in good shape.
- **From 2 to 3 seconds**: the pace is fast. It requires going over the same line several times to obtain a result. The effect is both relaxing and invigorating, as it stimulates the surface and the Yang energy. It is a very good rhythm to unclog mechanical and muscular problems.
- **From 3 to 5 seconds**: this rhythm is a good balance between Yin and Yang. It contacts the Blood level and balances the body and the mind while deepening the relaxation of the recipient.
- **From 5 to 12 seconds**: this slow pace stimulates the Yin energy to re-energize a tired person. It will contact the deep levels and activate the parasympathetic nervous system. It usually requires only one pass per work line.
- **More than 12 seconds**: we reach into what are called connections, whose purpose is to harmonize the energy between two *tsubos* ツボ (pressure points) or two meridians, or between the receiver and the practitioner. This often happens between two points of contact (both thumbs or palms of the hand).

If you want to be able to accomplish a Shiatsu adapted to each case that comes into your practice, it is interesting to master all these rhythms in the pressure and not to limit yourself to one way of proceeding. That is why we must always be wary of dogmas. In my classes I usually say, "If you have a paper fan open just slightly, when you wave it you will not have much air movement; the effect is almost nothing. If you open the fan completely, it will work much better." When Shiatsu training is done full-time,[2] the teaching reviews all the rhythms of pressure. Some schools go so far as to preserve the best of all styles and throw away the dogmas, in order to focus only on the therapeutic aspect. On humanitarian missions using Shiatsu, it is essential to know how to constantly adapt to everything that comes in, because you are far from the comfort of your practice and your usual clients. The cases are so varied that it is necessary to be able to quickly switch from one rhythm to another, depending on the person or the sensitivity of their body.

But this story of rhythm goes even further. One of the most competent teachers I have met in my *shiatsushi* life is Bernard Bouheret.[3] Author of many books, he has been living Shiatsu for more than 40 years. The biggest lesson one can receive from him is to watch him give treatment. Unlike Shiatsu styles with a unique rhythm, his varies regularly within the treatment. He speaks of it as a musical symphony. There is the introduction, the rise in power, then, as for a piece of music, ups and downs, quiet times, fast times, sorts of choruses, staccatos and then a smooth conclusion. The changes of pace are never abrupt. He does not jump from one to the other, which would create a disharmony that would disturb the recipient. No, he does all this in a continuous progression, as if driving over a hilly landscape. This notion of setting to music, and therefore automatically of rhythm, allows a great richness in the treatment and the ability to constantly adapt rhythm and depth according to the feeling of the hands. In this way, the receiver has the sensation of all his aspects being "explored". At the same time, this is a soothing and complete feeling, nothing seems to have been forgotten. Kobayashi Sensei, the senior instructor at Japan Shiatsu College in Tokyo, demonstrated a complete treatment in Brussels in 2014 during an international workshop. Without a word and for almost an hour, his hands roamed the body like a pianist, moving from one rhythm to another and pausing when necessary. As a practitioner, it is boring to follow the same rhythm during a whole session, while by varying the rhythms you can be a real conductor, writing your compositions, creating your own music.

Silences

In music as in poetry, in painting as in speech, what gives relief is not so much the rhythm as the silences at the right moments. The notion of silence is crucial. Knowing how to stop running the fingers in a Shiatsu is like icing on the cake. It is a breath, a pause between two sequences, which offers a moment of respite to both the recipient and the donor. In this period of time, nothing happens. The *shiatsushi* listens to the body, deepens the connection, while the *jusha* gathers his strengths or lets go even deeper. The right time to take a break depends on the ability to feel. If you find a pain, a point of tension, there is no point in insisting too much with the hope that everything will pass. Sometimes you have to know how to wait, listen, accompany the receiver in the infinitely small, in the subtle. Sometimes, this is where the culmination of an entire treatment is composed, as if one were at the apex of a mountain before descending from it.

The question which then arises is how long should we hold this pause? The balance is delicate, and once again you have to trust your instinct and your listening. If you do nothing for an hour, the person in your hands will wonder why they came. If you end the pause too quickly, you may miss out on something essential.

Kawada Sensei said that he sometimes held a pressure unmoving for 45 minutes, until life returned to the point that interested him. In general, wait until you feel a change, even slight, in the heat, blood circulation or muscle fibres. It is the signal that a process is under way. Wait a little longer to make sure the process continues and move on to the rest of your symphony.

Rhythm is therefore not just an intellectual idea but a founding principle of the Shiatsu technique, which makes it possible to vary the effects and create depth. Better yet, the practitioner can from time to time also find the pleasure of reworking only in one rhythm, no longer because that is all he knows, but because he has chosen it. With the variations of rhythms and pauses in a Shiatsu practice, there is something in it for all the actors of a session and they enter fully into the notion of pleasure: pleasure to be treated and pleasure to give.

Summary

1. There are many rhythms in Shiatsu pressure. You have to learn them all so you don't get stuck in a routine.
2. The rhythms allow different effects depending on the time given to the pressure.
3. Pauses allow you to breathe and give depth to the treatment.
4. Changes of rhythm allow the practitioner to express his way of being and healing, and to explore many aspects of the recipient.

5

Verticality

One might think that an upright posture in Shiatsu serves above all to look pretty and to give an air of professional seriousness that favourably impresses the entourage, teacher or client. This may be the case, but it is certainly not the main reason that makes proper spinal alignment a principle in itself. This verticality of the back allows first of all to keep it in good condition, to work the back muscles, to strengthen them and to avoid premature wear of the vertebral discs. In addition, this verticality makes it possible to completely open the rib cage as well as the abdomen, thus promoting deep and soothing breathing. The belly thus cleared, the hips can work, articulate, without being blocked.

Reflections about verticality

Man's greatest achievement, before fire, was to straighten up and walk on two legs. What may seem today as a given and completely trivial fact is in reality a revolution such that it still has profound repercussions in our lives. Changing from quadruped to biped took a few million years of evolution. It wasn't the case that one of our ancestors succeeded overnight. It took a long and patient adaptation of our skeleton and locomotor system. The first consequence of straightening is the widening of the pelvis, allowing us to stand and walk. Until then the pelvis was at the back of the body (the famous hindquarters). Now it is placed in the centre and separates the upper and lower body. The point of equilibrium is no longer at the stomach's *Bo* (or *Mu* in Chinese) point, but three fingers under the navel,[1] which considerably changes the situation, digestively and energetically speaking. Since then, the body has revolved around the pelvis, allowing lateral twists that were not possible before. This also moved the centre of sexual urges and the area of procreation up to the heart of our body. Mating can now be done face-to-face, with all the consequences we can imagine (looking into each other's eyes, expressing our feelings...). And that's not to mention raising the head thanks to the occipital hole, bringing the eyes closer together to allow us to see in front of us and in three dimensions, and so on.

The spine has undergone a great transformation in this process. Instead of being subject to the earthly attraction in its centre and bending downwards (think of the back of mammals), it becomes the framework that allows the body to stand straight, a role that previously was devolved to the four limbs. The spine became of crucial importance and equipped itself with a double curvature to allow it to absorb shocks without compacting all the vertebrae. With this upright posture, the skull grew considerably, the eyes could see further, and Man could anticipate dangers or obstacles and therefore – via his nervous system – manage the muscular effort he needed. If eyesight becomes important, the sense of smell decreases, and the nose loses its keenness. But above all, the feet flatten for walking and the hands are freed, permitting the grasping of objects and the creation of tools. It is often said that, without his hands, Man would be nothing and this is quite true, especially if we look at it from the point of view of Shiatsu.

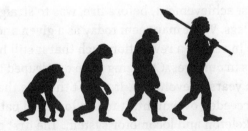

All this is only a brief overview of the profound changes that the human being has experienced with the vertical position and there is still much to say, especially at a muscular (the organs must protect themselves with the help of an abdominal barrier), physiological (the stomach that once digested lying flat is now upright) and energetic (Man finds himself making the link between Heaven and Earth) level.

Lack of verticality

Alas, despite these millions of years of efforts to straighten up, it is more than common to see students and even high-level practitioners bend their backs forward during Shiatsu. This lack of back position results in a whole set of postural imbalances that slow down or even prevent correct technique. By bending, the practitioner will tend to lower the head as well, which strains the muscles of the neck and tires the cervical vertebrae.

Another thing the practitioner should no longer need to constantly look where he puts his fingers to know what he is doing. The shoulders are hunched forward, which closes the top of the rib cage and prevents a good opening of the lungs. By bending the back forward, the rib cage blocks the abdomen, which in turn prevents the diaphragm from descending. Finally, constantly bending the column and in only one direction tends to make it pinch the discs, always on the same side (on the front edge).

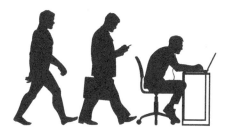

In the long run, this posture can lead to serious mobility problems of the trunk. In short, it is the whole anatomy of the practitioner that will have struggle with practising Shiatsu, on the one hand, and feeling the benefits and pleasure of the practice on the other hand. Students who do not respect the principle of verticality quickly get hurt and abandon Shiatsu, thinking that it is not for them. What a pity! This is why teachers are always right to demand good posture, so as not to let students spoil the fruit of millions of years of evolution.

Of course, this degradation of verticality is not the fault of students alone but of our entire so-called modern society. After the end of the Second World War, the world changed profoundly. Before that, most people worked in a standing position, whether in the fields, in factories or in crafts. Usually, they sat for three hours a day and stood for eight to nine hours. After the war, the situation was completely reversed in less than 50 years. With the arrival of a services-based society, then the arrival of computers, people spend most of their time sitting and barely two to three hours on their legs. Bodies grew (20 to 30 cm more in two generations) quickly and became less solid (weaker bones) thanks to less movement but also thanks to a weaker musculature. Think of a typical day for a Western city dweller: he gets up, then sits down for breakfast. He sits in transport to go to work where he sits for two periods of at least four hours. In between, he goes to lunch, sitting in a canteen or restaurant. In the evening, tired, he eats before collapsing on the sofa in front of the TV or his home computer. Then he lies down to sleep. The long hours in sitting postures bend the lower back, creating all kinds of lower back pain. As for the upper back, it goes forward so that the eyes can get closer to the screens. As a result, the back muscles, constantly supported by a chair, are no longer strong enough to hold the upright posture, and back problems have become a major disorder since the second half of the 20th century. During meditation classes, all beginners tell me the pain they have when they have to stay straight and motionless for more than ten minutes – only ten minutes. That is the situation we must face.

To drive (or to ram?) in the nail, smartphones continue to bending the neck forward, creating a multiplication of neck tensions and migraines. I've observed right angles in teenagers' necks, something that did not exist less than ten years ago. And it's obvious that the intervertebral discs are, from top to bottom, all pinched on their anterior surface and the legions of herniated discs that we see today emerging in 30-year-olds. The body knows how to adapt to new positions, but for this it takes at least a million years. We have changed our posture in less than 50 years, so our body is only at the beginning of this new phase of adaptation. We are not done with back pain. This is why it is essential to know how to maintain verticality.

Verticality and righteousness

The Japanese call the principle (and respect) of verticality *sei chu sen* (正中線). This term refers to the central line of the body, whether from the front or side, in its relationship with the point of balance of the body located in the *hara*. Beyond the correct attitude that it represents anatomically, verticality is also a moral, philosophical and energetic principle. Moral because the physical verticality induces, in the practitioner, a correct attitude towards the recipient. By straightening up, the practitioner will gradually have a better self-esteem in his work and the importance of his role in the support he offers to others. He becomes morally straight, without being stiff, like his backbone, which is straight yet remains flexible. To spin the metaphor, we can say that it is rare to meet terrorist yogis. The flexibility of the body almost automatically induces that of the mind, and the verticality of the body makes it possible to tend towards a higher level of consciousness.

According to the theory of Chinese medicine, Man is at the centre of a relationship between Earth and Heaven. Heaven and Earth represent his two horizons, but by its verticality he can (and for Shiatsu practitioners, he must) make the link between these two universes.

The mere fact that human beings stood up in the course of their evolution, puts Man in this position of moral and physical responsibility to make the link between Heaven and Earth. He is like a common thread that lets celestial and telluric energies pass through him. It is from this observation that the ancient Chinese found the channels of the meridians through which the energy of Heaven and Earth passes, in other words, *Ki* (in Japanese) or *Qì* (in Chinese).

Being straight and flexible at the same time allows good circulation of energy through the eight Extraordinary channels and the 12 meridians. But it is above all through the spine, a notion that is also found in India with the energy of the kundalini, that energy massively flows through the body. The column is like the heart of the trunk that is the human being, a line on which the seven chakras pulsate. In order to have a good flow of celestial energy through our body, this must not be blocked, twisted or, most importantly, suffer, or nothing can pass properly, and the *Ki* stagnates, dragging in its wake all kinds of symptoms. Energetically, so as not to exhaust ourselves and to convey it best to the receiver, it is necessary to let the Yin travel from Earth to Heaven and conversely the Yang from Heaven to Earth, all passing through us. Otherwise, the practitioner will draw from his reserves, tire and, finally, bend a little more towards the ground like the weeping willow.

Summary

1. Verticality is the result of a long evolution, its degradation the result of our modern life being spent essentially sitting.
2. Verticality makes it possible not to wear out the spine.
3. It strengthens the back muscles and keeps them in good shape.
4. It encourages the use of breathing and relaxation in the practitioner.
5. It paves the way for better self-esteem and morality, and the perception of one's role as a practitioner for other people.
6. Verticality is the only way to properly let the energy of Heaven and Earth pass through one's body.

6

Centring

The principle we discuss in this chapter is a little harder to grasp than the previous ones. In our society, we talk little about centring. We spend much of our time working our minds or staring at screens. Our energy is therefore essentially directed towards the brain, and we forget that we have a body. Now, to speak like the knight of Lapalisse, the centring is done in the centre, and not in the head. The peoples of Asia and the Indian subcontinent have always put the centre in the spotlight and, when they talk about centring, it is the abdomen that we are talking about. In Japanese, the *hara* is a very broad concept that encompasses a whole set of realities. It is the belly but also the centre of the individual, the centre of gravity, the digestive centre, the energy centre and the centre where the mind of the wise must be placed. For the record, Ananda, one of Buddha's most important disciples, asked: "Master, what is a wise man?" To which Buddha replied: "He is a man whose belly works well." This answer might make it seem that Buddha is gently mocking him, but this is not the case. The ability to live in one's centre is indeed the source of wisdom. This is why the wise men of the Far East are always represented with a round belly, sometimes enormous, to clearly indicate where their strength and wisdom reside.

Through the absorption, processing, transportation, digestion and elimination of food, we create energy that is quickly felt in the form of heat. All these physiological phenomena take place in the *hara*. These transformations will create *Ki*, which will then be distributed in the Three Burners, two of which are in the abdomen, then in the twelve meridians. The *hara* is therefore a factory for creating energy from food and mixing it with the air and the Essence of the Kidneys to make the true *Ki*.

On the importance of hara

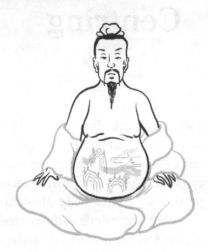

**THE BELLY IS THE SEAT OF THE CREATION
OF ENERGY AND SPIRITUAL LIFE.**

According to Asian teaching, all movements must spring spontaneously from the centre. Whether you are a sculptor, calligrapher, dancer, rice planter, swordsman or *shiatsushi*, there are no exceptions to this rule. Japan has taken this principle to its extreme with the samurai. Their way of walking was not the same as ours. Indeed, their arms did not follow their natural counterbalance movement but advanced at the same time as the leg of the same side.[1] Try walking with your left leg and left arm together, and then the same thing on the right, without feeling like you're out of balance. On the contrary, the purpose of this march was to not twist the trunk, but to constantly keep the *hara* straight through the hips and the right hand always parallel to the hilt of the sword, which was always facing the navel. Thus, the unsheathing of the sword was never troubled by an uncentring due to the twisting of the chest relative to the hips and the movement of the hand was always related to the *Ki* of the *hara*. Today, it would seem very complicated to walk in this way, but staying centred remains a crucial notion.

In Shiatsu the back-and-forth movement of the body starts from the belly, is to train practitioners to stay well centred in their belly. The movements are thus stable, calm, powerful and just. We have seen the importance of verticality to clear the *hara* and leave it free to breathe and fill. Abdominal breathing brings a movement of rise and fall to the diaphragm that relaxes and strengthens the internal organs of the practitioner, which brings a certain serenity in his life as in his work, if only because he is not constipated. The verticality of the body coupled with a soft and strong *hara* makes it easy to perform the rocking movement of the hips, which in turn offers enough power to exert the correct deep and painless pressure. To sum up, the application of pressure always and only starts from the *hara*, from the centre. Shiatsu cannot do without this work, on the one hand because it is a manual art from a precise Asian culture, and on the other hand because it brings many benefits to the practitioner.

The centring in the *hara* is also called anchoring. The notion then goes beyond the simple physiological process to cover a more psychological character. To anchor oneself is to strengthen one's mind and bind it firmly to the body. In Japanese this is called *chinkon* (鎮魂). This term means "calming of the mind". It is often associated with *kishin* (帰神), whose meaning is "return to the Divine", or more precisely, to the *Ki* of the spirits (*kami*). To anchor ourselves would therefore be to return to the Divine that is in us by calming the mind. Be that as it may, in all Japanese traditions, spiritual or martial, the individual seeks to increase his anchorage so as not to get carried away easily, to stay in touch and in balance between body and mind. *Chinkon* is therefore a double exercise that has the advantage of calming and becoming strong. When we speak here of strength, it is not muscular strength that we are talking about, but of the mind that does not let itself be disturbed and of the body that does not let itself be decentred. Thus, the Shiatsu practitioner is always at the centre of himself and at the centre of the world. He should not be surprised by what he hears or feels. He becomes the reference for the receiver.

From this arises the importance of caring for your belly and massaging it regularly. For this there are several very useful methods: auto-Shiatsu, Anpuku, *chineitsang* (or *qineizang*, which translates as "massage of the energy of the organs") or constant abdominal breathing. The Qìgōng of the Iron Shirt allows an even more intense strengthening of the *hara*, but it is necessary to meet a master capable of teaching this technique generally oriented towards its martial aspect. Continuous breathing in full consciousness is preferable as it has the advantage of not being expensive and creates an internal massage movement of the abdomen. It is of course also necessary to think about a healthy and easy-to-digest diet, without forgetting to cleanse one organ or another once a year (draining of the Gallbladder, detoxification of the Kidneys, etc.). If the intestines and all the organs of the belly are well maintained and flexible, health is much better, energy becomes abundant and back problems resolve themselves when they are of intestinal origin.

Furthermore, to enquire how someone is in the morning, the Japanese ask: *O genki desuka*,[2] or literally "how is the root of your *Ki*," how are your *hara*, belly and intestinal transit, but also the form in which they are more generally. To which (previously at least) someone would respond by giving many details on the condition of their stool, which represents the easiest way to judge the quality of one's *hara*. Today things have changed somewhat.

Centring techniques

To be centred in the *hara*, it is first necessary to unblock breathing so that it descends into the abdomen, until it becomes automatic. However, most people have high breathing, often because of stress and poorly regulated emotions. Meditation allows you to become more grounded in your body. Without moving, in *seiza* or lotus position, the practitioner will place his mind, his consciousness, a little below the navel, towards the *kikai* point (CV6, *Qìhǎi*, or Sea of Energy). By placing the mind in this part of the body, thoughts quickly diminish, the body fills with calm and quiet strength. Little by little, the body relaxes while remaining straight, as if it were melting from the head to the ground. The body then becomes heavier and heavier and seems to spread on the ground beyond physical limits, as if it obtained a wider base, a bit like becoming a pyramid.[3] This sensation lowers the centre of gravity and strengthens the *hara*. The calm that this meditation generates makes it possible to carry out a serene and powerful

Shiatsu session, without thought and yet with great lucidity, as if it were only the obvious continuation of the meditation.

But not everyone manages to meditate, whether from lack of time or lack of discipline. It is possible to perform many exercises to strengthen centring.

- The practice of Taichichuan (*Taijíquán*) reinforces the centring. This gentle martial art forces the practitioner to constantly reach the limits of his balance, then to make gestures without losing his balance. The slowness of the movement always leads the practitioner to feel the work in his centre. Experts of Taichichuan have such a powerful centre that they become impossible to uproot.
- In Shiatsu, there are many small exercises that are very useful, for example, sitting in *seiza* and rotating the body without lifting the knees or losing balance. At first, it seems difficult and the circle remains quite small. But with time and practice, the circle widens.
- It is also interesting to ask students to put their arms under another's armpits and to try to lift the one who is sitting. At first everyone seems to be light, but over time bodies are heavier and heavier. The simple relaxation of the belly and abdominal breathing help a lot.
- In my classes, I often ask a student to stand up and not move while another pushes him. Then a second person comes to help the first push, then a third, until the one who resists moves back. Progress from centring can be measured by the number of people needed to move the one receiving the push.
- In Aikidō, an exercise called *kokyu-hō* is often used. Two people face each other in *seiza* and one grabs both wrists of the other. The one who is seized must resist the thrusts of the other and not fall. As long as you use muscles, you will always end up falling over. As soon as you release tensions and use your belly, you become much more stable.
- Another Aikidō exercise is to place one student in *seiza* while the other person stands. The standing person pushes with both hands on the forehead of the sitting one.

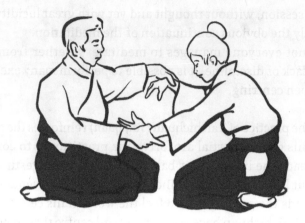

THE KOKYU-HŌ EXERCISE IS USED TO STRENGTHEN THE HARA.

- Finally, and to finish this small series of exercises, I propose that one student lies on his back. Another places both hands on his stomach and presses with all his weight. The student lying down must work with his belly, without contracting the abdominals, to lift the one above by the sole force of his abdominal breathing.

By making the link between the centre of the body, the centre of creation of energy, the centre of the Middle and Lower Burners, the centre of breathing, and the centre of the mind without thoughts (our famous second brain), we then understand the importance afforded to the *hara* and the notion of centring in Asian medicine. Centring increases mental strength, emotional stability and the depth of the gesture; in other words, centring gives presence. With such a presence, not only is the technical quality at the rendezvous, but the receiver can let go because he is taken care of by a strong and benevolent personality, without judgement. The regular practice of centring in the *hara*, whatever your favourite means, is always a winning bet for the success of a good Shiatsu.

Summary

1. Centring in the *hara* is the keystone of all the arts of Asian culture.
2. The *hara* is the centre of energy and of calmness of the mind.
3. Abdominal breathing and meditation strengthen centring.
4. A student should regularly practise *hara* strengthening exercises to learn how to centre.
5. A centred practitioner will be free of thoughts and possess a strong, benevolent and reassuring technique.

7

Continuous Breathing

First, last, outer, inner, only that
Breath breathing human being.

EXCERPT FROM THE POEM *ONLY BREATH*, BY RUMI

Since ancient times, man has been quick to understand the importance of correct breathing. Many traditions on all continents show
that very early in history, the breathing technique was deeply studied
to obtain different effects: more physical resistance (in China with
the Qìgōng of the Iron Shirt), more stamina (in Greece or Tibet with
running), more introspection in self-discovery (in India with meditation), more mysticism (all over the world and in all spiritualities),
more energy (Chinese Taoist breathing, in particular but not exclu-
sively). Obtaining so many different effects shows the importance of
the study of breathing. From the moment we are born and our first
inhalation, to the moment of our death and the last exhalation, our
whole life is conditioned by breathing. Its importance is paramount.

The Chinese have a proverb that says: "药补不如食补" (*Yào bǔ
bùrú shíbǔ*), which is: "Medicine is not as good as food." This means
that instead of seeking treatment, we must start by knowing what
we eat and pay attention to it. Oxygen is our first food. If we compare it with others, we quickly realize its importance. You daily eat
between 400 and 800 grams of solid food. It is possible to survive two
to three weeks without food. You drink one to one-and-a-half litres
of water every day to compensate the effects of sweating and urine
elimination. Without water, you can subsist for two or three days.
You breathe up to 12,000 litres of air a day and yet you wouldn't last

more than a few minutes without oxygen. These few figures make it possible to see how different their importance is. The more subtle the food, the more vital it is.

Three levels of breathing

The body breathes automatically, which does not mean that we breathe properly. To take a point of comparison, everyone knows how to run, but only those who are trained can run and break records. For breathing it is the same. It is therefore essential to learn how to breathe. The first thing to know about breathing is that it works on three levels.

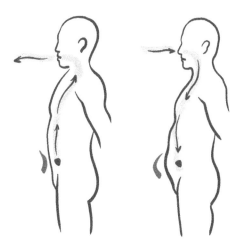

EXHALATION: THE BELLY GOES IN.
INSPIRATION: THE BELLY GOES OUT.

- **Top breathing**: from the nose to the chest, breathing is short and insufficient for good health.
- **Middle breathing**: from the nose to the diaphragm, without it going down properly. This is already better than the previous situation, but the lungs cannot fully develop due to the blocked diaphragm.
- **Low breathing**: breathing activates a back-and-forth movement of the abdomen, which indicates that the diaphragm is moving up and down freely. This breathing massages the

organs and viscera, softens the entire belly, facilitates bowel movement, allows the lower spine to move and activates the production of energy from the Kidney.

It is obvious that the deeper and more relaxed the breath, the better the body is oxygenated. This notion is crucial. Indeed, the brain alone consumes about 20 per cent of the oxygen you breathe, yet it represents only 2 per cent of the human body weight. The same goes for nutrients, 20 per cent of which end up in the brain. This distribution of resources is not at all equal, to say the least. However, as soon as you breathe deeply and quietly, the brain meets with an abundance of oxygen that irrigates and relaxes it automatically. Your mind is calmer, thinks less and therefore requires less oxygen. As a result, the rest of the body will benefit from an additional supply of oxygen in the blood, and will avoid having to breathe heavily, making a noise during a Shiatsu, which always disturbs the recipient. You have probably already received a Shiatsu with a person who starts to breathe noisily or to blow on your face... It's rather unpleasant, isn't it?

Breathing and health

To mark the importance of breathing for our daily health, I explain this to my students as to my recipients:

- If you breathe, you are alive.
- If you are not breathing, you are dead; so far it is logical.
- But if you breathe well, you are or will be healthy.
- So, if you breathe poorly, you are or will be sick.

Health depends a lot on the quality of breathing. If breathing is blocked, the person feels bad, lacks oxygen, feels tightness in the chest, worry or even anxiety; his body tenses, the brain works less well. This short list of side effects is probably the best way to spot the emergence of one symptom or another in a fairly short time. It can be said that the terrain is not good and will weaken, opening an easy road for any sort of physical illness or psycho-emotional disorder. If you are not convinced, do the following test: bend your back and block the diaphragm, close your shoulders forward and try to breathe properly. You will quickly feel oppressed, and if you observe your psyche over 10 to 20 minutes, you will experience a decrease in vigour. After an hour, the first negative ideas will inevitably arrive. From there, the whole body–mind–set will slowly worsen. Emotions are directly influenced by breathing, especially because in Chinese medicine it is said that their centre is in the chest, at point CV 17 precisely (*Danchū* 膻中, middle of the chest). Now reverse the process, open the shoulders, inflate the chest, inhale deeply through the nostrils and you feel your body open, become conquering, and your mind regains its good feelings.

The other important aspect of breathing is that it must be done continuously. However, a large number of people experience breaks in this entirely natural process. At a time of intense concentration – writing, listening to an important conversation, in the presence of an invasive or aggressive person (in French, we say "il me pompe l'air"[1]), worrying about a child or a parent – many people block their breathing. Add to this all the nighttime breathing disorders, such as the famous sleep apnea which is relatively common, and you will understand that many people suffer from poor breathing, and consequently, poor oxygenation. For the Shiatsu practitioner, continuous breathing is the tool that precedes the action of his fingers. When he is next to the receiver, he starts by calming down and feeling his body. To do this, he checks that his breathing is ample, calm and continuous. He thus ensures that he will not be disturbed by it during the session and will not find himself short of breath if he has to make an effort or two.

To return to health and breathing, we now know that two phenomena are at the root of the degradation of our cells: acidification of our body fluids and oxidative stress. The latter is a combination of lack of water and lack of oxygen. Cells live and function thanks to these two essential elements for life. Many people, and this is always a source of surprise for a practitioner like me, do not like to drink water and prefer coffee and sodas. The body lacks water and its acidity skyrockets. Coupled with the lack of oxygen, cells weaken, die or mutate. This process is recognized today as one of the causes of the development of cancer cells. Add processed sugar, very present in industrial food, and the deteriorated cells will grow at high speed. Breathing is therefore one of the basic keys to our health.

Mindful breathing

To improve breathing as much as possible, it must be done mindfully. As in meditation, it is necessary to let go of bodily mechanisms (do not force anything). It must also be deep and relaxed to avoid internal tensions and continue the auto-massage of the organs in order to release good energy from the Three Burners. This is the basis of the making of Ki. However, one of the most common problems that we see among students is apnea. These apneas are not done consciously. They occur when the *shiatsushi* performs a difficult movement, or a physical effort; the difficulty is to become aware of it. To become aware does not mean to think about it constantly, but to be permanently aware of what is happening in oneself. In short, you should not have to think about your breathing but be alerted as soon as it does not go well. This is the secret to mindfulness of everything that is happening in our body as well as in our mind.[2]

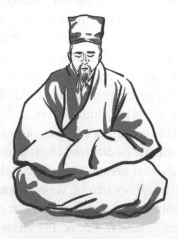

DEVELOPING POWER THROUGH BREATHING.
TAOISTS CALL THIS NEI GŌNG 内工, MEANING "INNER WORK".

If your breath is cut off at regular intervals, your body will run out of oxygen, then take deep breaths and exhalations to compensate. You then fall back into the trap of loud breathing and disturbing noise, not to mention small cardiac accelerations to regulate the distribution of oxygen by the blood. In addition, you create an intermittent, even chaotic energy, which will not physically help you to give several sessions in the same day. This is why it is essential that breathing is automatically continuous and smooth. The Japanese call this principle *kokyū ryoku* (呼吸力). If *kokyū* alone can be translated as "breath", the combination of the two words will place more emphasis on the notion of breathing power. This expression shows that mechanically breathing is the result of an inhalation and an exhalation in a continuous cycle that produces energy. Furthermore, in Japanese, the word for the great universal energy is *Tai kokyū* (太呼吸), which means "the great breath".

The practitioner sets the pace

The Shiatsu practitioner is, for his patient, not only a person of knowledge and technical skills, but also an example in terms of health and quality of being. The way he breathes must be an example for the recipient's body. Without a word, the way you breathe becomes the model for the receiver. There is a good reason for this. If someone comes to see you, it is because they are not well. In this case, we cannot rely on the quality of his breathing rate. This is why the practitioner does not have to follow the pace of the recipient's breathing but works to his own pace. In other words, he embodies the standard of correct breathing, the one that must be followed. The recipient's body will gradually model itself on yours and breathe at your rhythm. This requirement to be a model for the other is difficult, which is why a *shiatsushi* must regularly work on himself and remain as attentive during a Shiatsu session as in his daily life. This permanent work of improving, following a high goal, serving as an example for his clients, shows that Shiatsu is not just a technique, but a Way to follow all one's life.

Better yet, the practitioner's breathing helps establish the standard for pulse rate. During one inhale-exhale, we must be able to count, on average, four beats of the client's pulse. The pulse is taken by counting the beats in relation to the practitioner's breathing. This shows how much his breathing must be of a good quality. Therefore, he must regularly practise breathing exercises to improve it, self-massage his abdomen, do meditations to deepen and relax it, become aware of his breathing so as not to disturb the recipient, and observe the quality of his breathing to become a reference for his client.

Having said that, there are exceptions to the rule that the practitioner follows his breathing rhythm and not that of his client. In some cases, it is useful to use (not follow) the inhale and exhale of the *jusha* to perform certain pressures. These pressures accompany the exhalation and aim to go deep into the body to obtain relaxing effects or to expel air from the rib cage. But during a session, this is rather a technique, a short passage, to obtain a desired effect. Once this technical moment has passed, the practitioner returns to his own pace and becomes the reference again.

When working in energetics, the practitioner also tunes into the breathing of the recipient. This time it's about something else. The practitioner's body becomes the receptacle of a need, an unconscious request on the part of the recipient. It is no longer he who follows his own rhythm, but it is the Breath – in the sense of *Qì* – that requires him to get in tune to help the person. It is said that the practitioner is not breathing: he is breathed. Breathed by something bigger than him that takes control at this precise moment. This moment is very important to observe because it is usually then that blocked situations are resolved. This often results in an acceleration of breathing in case of stagnations, or slowing down in psycho-emotional disorders. Once the receiver's block is lifted, everyone resumes their rhythm.

While we are talking about the practitioner's breathing, it seems important to me to speak of a curious but quite common phenomenon: metabolization. It happens quite often – during or after a treatment – that a practitioner starts to burp or hiccup. This can be quite embarrassing for the receiver, but in fact it is a completely natural principle. The key is to warn him at the beginning of the session if this tends to happen for you. When the receiver frees himself of energy nodes, the practitioner receives the overflow and metabolizes it in the form of air bubbles that obviously seek to get out, hence the burps. The underlying mechanism is not yet fully understood, but it should not worry students. The teacher will be there to explain other ways to evacuate energy discharges or how to discreetly manage these unwanted noises.

Summary

1. Continuous breathing provides a constant source of energy.
2. It avoids apneas, and hard or noisy breathing in the practitioner.
3. Breathing must be deep and relaxed, to avoid tension and oxygenate the whole body-mind.
4. Breathing should take place mindfully.
5. Properly managed, breathing becomes the reference for taking the pulse of the recipient.

8

Two Hands Together

If traditionally, in Japan, Anma massage was reserved for blind practitioners,[1] it was not intended for armless practitioners! Indeed, to do a good massage it is better to use both hands to maximize the effects. This is even truer for Shiatsu. Both hands work together in all cases. Let's take the example of stretching. To avoid using strength while holding, use both hands and shift the weight of the body while relaxing the muscles from the shoulders to the wrists. If you hold with one hand, the grasp is likely to slip. Or you are holding a limb (leg or arm) in each hand, which rebalances the traction on two identical supports. In the case of stretching, two-handed work is always a plus, but this is also true for the entire technical catalogue.

Now imagine that you are trying to mobilize a joint that is a bit rigid, such as the shoulder. Again, both hands work together, otherwise you will have little impact on the shoulder. Or one serves as a support, a fixed point, while the other moves the joint. This mobilization work against a static resistance often makes it possible to open the joint further. Or you can use both hands together to have a little more power in a rotational movement, for example.

Of course, if you choose to make an energetic connection between two *tsubos*, you need both hands. The very principle of the connection is to let both hands or thumbs come into contact with each other through the body of the *jusha*. Like two poles of the same battery, the hands will always manage to create a flow of energy and connect through the body of the recipient, regardless of their respective positions. It may take more or less time, but in any case, by working together, it is possible to do a lot with this simple technique.

Benefits of working with two hands

From experience, I know that forgetting to work with two hands usually occurs when the student or practitioner approaches technical movements or begins to think about the location of the points, a flaw that can be seen especially in therapeutic Shiatsu. Since it is a question of using points that are chosen to respond to a specific pathology, why not use only one thumb? This is an easy way, certainly, but it is a big mistake for several reasons.

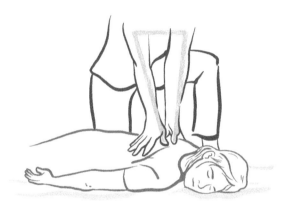

HERE WE SEE NOT ONLY THE TRIANGULATION OF THE FORCES IN ACTION BUT ALSO THE CIRCULATION OF ENERGY THAT GOES FROM ONE THUMB TO THE OTHER THROUGH THE CHEST AND THE HEART.

- First of all, two thumbs will do a more efficient and less tiring job than one, which may wear out in the long term. With two thumbs, you respect the triangle of pressure that forms with the torso.
- Second, the flow of energy is always better between two points of contact, whether they are the thumbs, fingers or palms. This also works with the elbows or soles of the feet.
- Finally, if only one thumb is apparently working, putting a hand further away makes it possible to listen to the reactions of the body, especially of the worked area, the muscle, the organ or the meridian.

The combined work of both hands therefore represents a vector of mechanical force, but this is not the only benefit. It is also the best way to multiply the possibilities. Among all the existing Shiatsu styles, Ohashiatsu requires practitioners to perform pressure work with one hand and stretching movement with the other, on a regular rhythm, for the entire session or close to it. This combination is very pleasant to receive because it stimulates the *tsubos* to achieve a real treatment whilst relaxing the sympathetic nervous system using a rocking technique.[2] We can clearly see here the potential of working with two hands.

Mother hand / daughter hand

If until now you are used to using only one hand, ask yourself what it would feel like if you were the recipient. Wouldn't you have the feeling of being only half touched? Two hands give a comforting sensation and allow you to let go, since the practitioner takes care of you completely. Thus, we return to the notion of presence that we mentioned earlier. Try to place the hand that is not used for pressure on the recipient's body. At first you put it anywhere, which is already pretty good. But if you can choose where, it will be even better, for example on the organ that corresponds to the meridian you are treating. The hand thus placed is not lifeless, quite the contrary. It will naturally connect with the area that is immediately within reach. From your palm you diffuse heat and energy and, for this reason alone, the receiver will thank you. Very often at the end of a session it is not uncommon to hear him say: "I do not know what you did, but your hands are warm, present, it's a pleasure."

Better yet, even a still hand, if properly placed and well connected, will turn into an ultra-sensitive stethoscope. It will become your eyes and ears, listening to the slightest changes that take place inside the recipient. This technique was popularized by the master Shizuto Masunaga, who called it "mother hand / daughter hand": one works while the other is passive, alternating roles. The passive hand remains attentive to the sensations of the body. The changes that it listens for are multiple: changes in temperature, tone, muscle tension and even vibration of the energy that circulates below. By working with both hands, you will find that the one that moves the least becomes the most essential. It reassures, it heats, it radiates, it connects and brings information from the bottom of the body and mind to your consciousness. Over the years, practitioners are surprised by the amount of intuitive information they perceive about the patient's condition, history, emotions, etc. This is all information that will help you better understand him and better help him relieve his problems.

Hands: Symbol of man

We can't talk about hands without speaking of the symbolism it represents. Without harmonious work between two hands, it would not have been possible for man to become a craftsman, to carve wood, to plant a nail or to tie a rope. And if writing has long been the prerogative of one hand, this period is over with the arrival of computers. Human work is always the fruit of his two hands. In addition, having a light, fast and powerful hand, and a heavy, deep and attentive hand is a beautiful representation of Yin and Yang. Our two hands are like the two aspects of the Chinese symbol that we value so much: a complementary duality that opens to all dualities as to the most essential unity.

Traditionally in Asia, when presenting an object or giving a gift, it is always held out with both hands, even if it is a simple business card. In the same way, one extends both hands to receive a gift or diploma from the hand of one's teacher. It is unthinkable not to offer and receive with all one's heart and therefore with two hands. Things are not half done in Asia when the act partakes a symbolic force. It is the same with the Taoist salute and the Buddhist salute; even the Christians' praying is done palm against palm.

It is also with both hands that we hold a baby to carry it. It is again with two hands that we support the child learning to walk. It is with two hands (and two arms) that one hugs someone who is suffering or crying, to console him. These last three sentences are not without analogy to Shiatsu, which seeks to relieve and help people. This is why the suffering person who comes to you for Shiatsu deserves no less than your two hands.

Summary

1. Working with two hands allows for more technical effects and contact with the recipient.
2. Even a motionless hand performs many beneficial actions: energy connection, heat source, sensitive radar that picks up information.
3. The two-handed technique is called "mother hand / daughter hand".
4. Two hands together increase the feeling of presence and care by the *shiatsushi*.
5. Two hands are the symbol of Yin and Yang in Shiatsu.

9

The Tools of the Body

In the official definition of Shiatsu in Japan, in 1955, the legislator endorsed the technique that defines Shiatsu by asserting three points:

1. Use of bare hands (no tools, elbow, knee or foot, etc.).
2. Body surface pressures (no rubbing, hitting or pushing).
3. The goal is to maintain and improve health or recover from illness.

But over time, many branches of Shiatsu have brought in the use of other parts of the body, while respecting the non-use of tools. This started both with Shizuko Yamamoto's "Barefoot Shiatsu" and with practitioners returning to Anma texts to understand the origins of Shiatsu. In Anma, many body tools are used and their influences are felt today, especially outside Japan. In Yoseidō Shiatsu for example, it is not uncommon to use elbows.

Let's see which body tools complement the basic technique.

The other fingers

Yubi 指

It's not just with the thumbs that the *shiatsushi* exerts pressure. The other fingers can also be used. For example, if you are above the head of a receiver lying on his back, it will be easier to press the BL1 and BL2 points with the index finger. If the index finger lacks power (it is not as strong as the thumb), the middle finger is superimposed on it to strengthen it. This way of doing things is quite classic in Shiatsu. In some schools, pressure is distributed between the five fingers of one hand. The desired effect is a wider diffusion of pressure, to relax a large muscle for example. You can also use your fingers to hook a muscle, to play it like a guitar string. This movement is found in Namikoshi's *kata* during work on the calf. In fact, one can easily use the index or middle finger to make energy connections, and after a few years of experience, it is possible to do it with any finger.

The palm

Tenohira 手のひら

The palm is the best-known tool for beginners in Shiatsu. It makes it possible to apprehend large areas, to examine them while exerting a first pressure. Beginners discover this tool before learning how to use the thumbs correctly, because the risk of hurting with the palms is quite low. In addition, the centre of the palm makes superb energy connections possible and/or warms the recipient's body. It is also possible to vary the angle of the hand and choose, for example, to press more with the heel of the hand, its cutting edge (hypothenar eminence) or the thenar eminence (muscular part under the thumb). This significantly changes the firmness of the pressure and its accuracy.

The fist

Ken 拳

Working with a closed fist is possible in Shiatsu, and it is interesting to use it, especially on the back when it is a little too stiff to work with the thumbs. In other words, it is good to relax the muscles to allow access to the *tsubos*. This greatly eases the work and avoids straining and wearing out the thumb joints. Furthermore, it is possible to vary the work with the fist. Do not close your fingers too much and the pressure of the fist will be relatively flexible. Close your fist like a stone and the pressure becomes more incisive, harder too. In other forms of massage therapy, especially using oil, one can see movements that twist the fist, with particular emphasis on the phalanges. In short, there are many ways of working with the fist. In Shiatsu, we keep with a perpendicular pressure, but with the power that comes from one or two fists, it is good to ensure that the receiver releases breath with each pressure and accompanies the movement. But the fist can also be used for percussions, a very pleasant technique to receive especially on the back or the sacrum. The only difference is that you do not close your fist (leave an opening in the centre of it) and have a supple wrist. So you can quickly and painlessly hit the back or any other part of the body capable of supporting this technique. Personally, I also use *kento*, the bump formed between the back of the hand and the base of the fingers when the fist is closed, or the joint of the first phalanx. To sum up, the fist is a tool that can be used in many ways. It should therefore not be neglected.

The forearm

Zenwan 前腕

There are many areas that can be worked on with the entire forearm, including the back, but also the shoulders, glutes or thighs. For example, to free a person from false sciatica, you need to work powerfully on the inner and outer sides of the thigh. Given the size of an athlete's thigh, it is better to have a tool capable of working such muscle mass, a role that the fingers alone cannot undertake without harming yourself. The forearm can also be used at different angles, which completely changes the feeling for the recipient. The muscles of the underside of the forearm create long, diffused and relatively gentle pressure. With the topside, the pressure becomes stronger due to the presence of bones (radius and ulna) under the surface of the skin. With a sharp edge, the ridge of the ulna offers sharper work. It is up to you to decide according to the resistance of the tissues, the degree of pain felt by the recipient and the needs of the treatment.

The elbow

Hiji 肘

The elbow is also appreciated in Shiatsu, but it is by far the most powerful tool of the human body, so it is necessary to know how to use it and not to do so lightly because of the risk of generating significant pain. Folding the arm causes the olecranon to poke out clearly and this results in a sharp and piercing tool, much wider than a thumb. Its capacity to penetrate tissues is considerable, so you must not collapse on the recipient, and be aware of sensations so as not to hurt.

By extending the arm at a right angle it is possible to flatten the elbow and use the forearm at the same time. This is a simpler and less risky technique to use at first. It combines the power of the elbow with the wide squashing effect of the forearm. This technique is very useful, especially on the QL (quadratus lumborum) muscle. Bending the arm brings out the tip of the elbow, which makes it possible to work the *tsubos*, in a rather large but penetrating way. Again, it is possible to do fluidic Shiatsu. I remember Master Kawada insisting that one must be able to bring out the *Ki* from the elbows and knees and to be just as effective as with the fingers or the palm. So, worth a try.

The knee

Hiza ひざ

Another joint of the body, rounder than the elbow but larger, the knee requires a good control of the *tate hiza* and *iai goshi* postures. These make it easy to raise and lower a knee and move it. Kawada Sensei, founder of Yoseidō Shiatsu, showed in his classes how to use the knee on almost all parts of the body. The difficulty lies in the balance – and therefore the stability – of the practitioner, who is deprived of one of his supports on the ground. This is why the work of balance must often be compensated by resting the hands on the body. Do not put pressure with the knee on a thigh, for example, without being perfectly sure of your stability in the movement. In case of loss of balance, you will literally crush the receiver. The knee is one of the less loved tools of the body, partly for its lack of precision, and practitioners prefer the elbow. All the same, train with the knee, in order to vary the use of your body and to be able to react to all situations. As Kawada Sensei said: "Imagine yourself facing a sumo. What would you do?" Masunaga, Ohashi, Bouheret and many others all show techniques with the knees, especially on the QL, the glutes or the back of the thigh.

The foot

Ashi 足

Here is another example of a body tool that is not appreciated enough. For their part, Ayurvedic or Thai masseurs do not hesitate to use their feet, even if it means walking on the back of the recipient, but in the Chinese and Japanese traditions it is rarer. In Shiatsu, the foot is not used enough, yet it conceals many possibilities. Yamamoto Sensei was the only one to put it in the spotlight in Shiatsu in a book that is still a reference[1] and taught, among others, by the Canadian professor Stéphane Vien. This resulted in a style known as A-shiatsu. In Kōhō Shiatsu, in the Omiya dojo, foot techniques are also numerous. Massaging the sole of the recipient's foot with the feet of the practitioner is a classic. The foot can be used flat, on its edge, with the heel, and we can even add working with a bent big toe to apply pressure, on the first point of the Kidney for example. The foot can also be used to block an area in a stretch, such as the armpit, while stretching the arm, or the square of the back to stretch the psoas, etc.

Tools of the body: Common features

In all cases, we must not waver from the rules of pressure without force, posture and verticality, all these essential aspects that set up and define the Shiatsu technique. When using these body tools, you must also pay more attention to what you press, because the areas are wider and sometimes it is possible to accidentally crush a fragile area. Think about working the back with the elbow flat. If you press on the spine, pain will soon appear, and the recipient will make a face. It is therefore necessary to stay on the muscles and, for this, to know them well. Shiatsu is a pressure technique that is practised through a sheet or clothes. Under no circumstances is massage oil used. When you see in some places proposals of Shiatsu with oil, I have only one piece of advice: pass it by. The mixing of genres is rarely successful. Furthermore, no additional tools should be used. This is found in Thai massage or Tok Sen,[2] but not in Shiatsu. Only body tools are allowed. We can say that it is a 100 per cent human technique.

Another aspect not to be ignored: the energetic dimension. You should not neglect the energy flow at the point of contact just because you are using a tool other than the thumbs or palms of your hands. A practitioner must be able to direct his energy anywhere in his body when working with it, whether it is the elbow, the foot or the fist. Admittedly, some places of the body are less easy to contact and energize, such as the knee, but this is mainly due to lack of habit and exercise. The use of body tools thus becomes a good way to get out of your automatisms. Yes, you probably already know how to send energy from the palms or thumbs, but you have been doing it by dint of work since the beginning of your studies. The fingers and palms learned to feel, developed a large number of skin sensors under the skin (Mesmer's corpuscles, Pacini's, etc.), then concentrated and released energy from there. Why? Because you've always worked with those parts of the body. Practise with the other tools regularly and you will gradually find the same abilities to feel, focus an intention and release an energy flow. There is nothing impossible about this but it involves work, work and more work.

Summary

1. The body includes many tools for pressing: finger, palm, forearm, elbow, knee and foot. Do not ignore them; do not settle for only one or two telling yourself that is enough.
2. Each tool of the body is used differently; you have to study them. But all of them require strict respect of the principles seen earlier, especially stability, verticality and the absence of strength in perpendicular pressure.
3. The use of body tools other than fingers and palms does not mean that we should forget about energy. We must feel it in every one of them. This takes practice.

10

Empathy

Your child has just fallen off his bike; you rush to hug him and help him up. Your best friend just went through a break-up; you listen to them and comfort them as they cry. A suffering parent is hospitalized for a serious illness; you go to their bedside to bring them support and comfort. In all these cases – and many more – you show empathy. This principle is at the heart of our human behaviour (even other mammals know this feeling), and without empathy, humanity would have destroyed itself long ago.

Empathy and compassion

Empathy comes from the Greek *empatheia* (εμπαθεια), from the Greek word *empathes* (εμπαθης), meaning "affected, who is passionate, exposed to the passions, sickly", itself derived from the prefix *en* (εν) and *pathos* (παθος) meaning "what one feels, state of a soul agitated by external circumstances, moral disposition, what happens to someone, endured experience". The term "compassion" comes from the Latin *cum patior* and literally means "to suffer with". So, it's the same thing. This may seem strange because today people no longer use these words with the same meaning as those indicated by their roots. Indeed, a semantic shift has taken place over time and the word "empathy" has taken on the meaning of "feeling what the other feels". In the therapeutic environment (psychological or physical), empathy has become a virtue that allows the practitioner to support and to accompany a person in his transformation process. The word "compassion" found itself locked into the lexical field of religion, thus allowing the two words to follow a different trajectory in the English language. However, under no circumstances should the practitioner suffer with his patient. He is not asked to do so. Never. If you wish to embark on the path of compassion, I recommend that you go to work in Calcutta in the Mother Teresa hospices; it is the best possible school for exercising compassion. When you study Buddhist meditation, you will also be told about compassion for oneself, then for others, and finally for all living beings. But in the therapeutic context, this is not what is asked of you from your teachers or even from the person who comes to see you.

The risk of confusing the meanings of empathy and compassion can take you quite far. First of all, psychologically, you may start bearing the cases of your patients outside the session and start ruminating on them. I think you already have enough to carry in your own psycho-emotional backpack, and other family baggage attached to it. No need to burden yourself with those of others. Energetically speaking, you create openings that do not need to be, and you put yourself in a position of weakness. The energy of the recipient's suffering will find its way into you through these weaknesses. Quickly, you will feel the physical pain of the patient, his physiological disorders, and really end up suffering with him. The patient will not necessarily be relieved. This case is much more common than you may think, especially when you start in Shiatsu. So do not play the part of a sponge, and maintain a healthy distance that allows you to be empathetic but not compassionate. If a word or situation of your patient makes you react emotionally, it is because it resonates within you. You will have to work within yourself on this aspect so that there is no more resonance. In this case, the help of an advanced teacher or psychotherapist as part of a supervision will greatly help you.

The impulse of the heart

What exactly is empathy? It is not a reaction of the body or the psyche. It is the impetus of a good and solid heart, which welcomes a person and helps him to get over a step in his life. In other words, empathy is an action, not a reaction to a situation. "Welcoming" is the correct term in the therapeutic relationship. You can have empathy in your daily life, but you will not go to all the suffering people you meet in the street to offer them Shiatsu, otherwise you will be quickly overwhelmed, and your behaviour would not be well perceived! Empathy in a therapeutic relationship means not being insensitive to what the patient feels, being able to accept him as he is and to put your technical skills at his disposal to help him.

Help him, okay... But to do what exactly? You can set yourself the goal, not to remove all forms of physical or psychological pain – this is not possible, a *shiatsushi* is not a superman or a superwoman – but rather to help him by accompanying him within the limits of your means, the Shiatsu technique. It is very important to remember that you have an obligation of means (hence initial studies of at least three or four years, work on oneself and continuing education) but not of results (otherwise you will experience Shiatsu as a great frustration). Empathy therefore makes it possible to show the person where they are, to make them aware by touch and sometimes by judicious life advice of their difficulties, blockages and suffering parts that they often ignore. You are not there to analyse this, leave that to the therapists. Empathy also allows you to show them different paths for progress and to designate the best one, but without forcing or imposing your point of view. Empathy finally makes it possible to accompany the patient on the path he or she has chosen, which is not necessarily the one you thought would be the most effective or the shortest but the one that will be the best for them at that time. This accompaniment means that you walk with the person, but you do not carry them (especially outside of working hours), because you will always lose that game.

To fully understand the feeling that guides the empathy of the practitioner, we must reread the maxim of Tokujiro Namikoshi that states: *Shiatsu no kokoro hahagokoro* ("Shiatsu is like the heart of a mother", implied "for her child"). This line of conduct, written by one of the four great founders of Shiatsu, is still learned by heart in all schools of this style, starting with the Japan Shiatsu College in Tokyo, the oldest and largest training centre in the world. The students recite it at every opportunity, they even made a song out of it. Thus, we understand that the essence of Shiatsu is a movement of the heart commonly called "universal love". This universal love is the ability to recognize oneself in the other, regardless of one's social or ethnic origins, convictions, gender or age. Shiatsu is a reflection of this ability. Better, it is its physical translation. Just like a child who is in pain after a fall from a bike, the practitioner takes the *jusha* like a mother, picks him up little by little, dries his tears, with patience restores his confidence in his abilities and relaunches him in life.

Empathy and resonance

Empathy opens your Heart to another's suffering, without it becoming yours, but at least you can feel what he is undergoing. It is an opening between you and the other, a connecting point, a stretched rope. This is called resonance. When the empathetic connection is established, you can do an incredible thing: put yourself in the other person's shoes. Not intellectually, but physically and emotionally. So, you feel in your body their knots and sufferings, and sometimes it shakes you strongly, as in this haiku of Soseki:

Over the wintry
forest, winds howl in rage
with no leaves to blow.

And yes, the storm rages, but you have within you the ability to extend a helping hand. It's easier to let yourself be guided when you feel the information coming from the other. No matter what issue you're working on, empathy is a first-rate tool to help your recipient.

I can give you two cases that, a priori, have nothing to do with each other and that I treated: a young girl who had bedwetting problems, and a widow who could not mourn her husband, a year after his death.

In the first case I was looking for what was wrong with the girl and the whole session went very well without me being able to distinguish a significant imbalance that would have allowed me to follow a track, a meridian or even a point. Suddenly, I realized that I was acting like a doctor and that I had forgotten the importance of resonating with her. After a few minutes, the empathy I felt with her allowed me to say, "Actually, everything is fine with you, isn't it?" The girl approved, she felt perfectly fine. This is how we discovered together that her disorder was not her problem but that of her parents. I then asked the mother to come and receive a Shiatsu at the next session, then to have a serious discussion with her husband about the image they conveyed to their child. The girl had no more problems from that day on.

In the second case, the widow, in her early sixties and a little plump, had not been able to cry at the death and burial of her husband. And after a year, she felt something was wrong. I did not ask why, but I simply put my hands on her stomach and chest with all the empathy in the world in the face of the distress she must be feeling, because if we do not cry at the death of one loved for a lifetime, then when? The hand on the heart indicated a tightening of the chest and the one on the stomach gave me the image of a cool cloud that stagnated there, between the skin and the muscles. This is of course anatomically impossible. I asked her if she wanted to bring out this cloud of tears and some time later, when she was ready, I massaged both the belly and the chest, while opening the Cloud Door (Lu 2) in connection with PC 6. She cried for three days straight. After that, her first action was to remove the portraits of her husband from the walls of her house. The grieving process was finally under way.

If there is no empathy, you cannot resonate and find what the person needs. But empathy does not mean that we will protect the person from their own suffering. On the contrary, we will guide her with delicacy to confront her demons, whether it is pleasant or not. This is the whole principle of therapy. But a therapy that is done by and for the heart, without the need to analyse the why and how. Empathy is our strongest weapon with which to physically touch the recipient and reassure him at the same time. We are all human. Let's use our best means of communication, our most beautiful language: that of the heart.

On the road to joy

But finally, what is the use of this empathy, this impulse of the heart that we are talking about here? A means of communication certainly, but towards what or rather towards what state of being? As we learn in class, the Heart is the home of a particular emotion: joy. But not the joy of having won the lottery, or laughing at a good pun, even if that is also undoubtedly pleasant. No, we are talking about this incredible and deep joy that makes us vibrate and makes us say: "I love life!" For of all the organs that manage emotions, not only do the Heart and joy have a direct relationship, but it is said in the classical texts that only the Heart feels all emotions. It is therefore a crossroads that is both terrible and exciting. And that's not all. To finish this small list, the Heart is the home of the Spirit (Shén).

Around us, we see so many people whose Hearts are wilting. Their Hearts have suffered too much, they are too heavy, they are no longer lively and bouncy as when one is a child. And yet it is the children who are right to be enthusiastic about everything, to laugh and shout with joy for the slightest thing. But over time... Through empathy we touch the Heart of the recipient. And if our practitioner's Heart is full and happy, then we can revive the extinguished Heart, give it back the spark of primary joy. It must never be a metronome of passing time, like an old clock abandoned in a corner. The Heart beats for the joy of living, to give joy to the spirit and to become again a child amazed and happy with this incredible gift that has been given to him: a body for playing and discovering. I can only encourage you to find this ability within yourself to transmit it through your soul, your words and your Shiatsu. That's why, like it or not, Shiatsu is not a simple technique, but an extraordinary tool to give joy back to people.

This is probably the greatest care that can be given. So let's end this chapter with these words of the great poet Tagore:

> *When old words die out on the tongue,*
> *new melodies break forth from the heart;*
> *and where the old tracks are lost,*
> *new country is revealed with its wonders.*[1]

Summary

1. Empathy is never to be confused with compassion, especially in a therapeutic relationship, ensuring that you do not suffer.
2. Empathy is a movement of the heart, like a mother's heart for her child when he suffers.
3. Empathy allows the patient to work with kindness, accuracy and attentiveness, then guides the patient to a solution that suits him.
4. Shiatsu is the technical translation of the empathic principal and allows you to resonate with the receiver.
5. The purpose of empathy is to resurrect joy in hearts.

11

The Different Techniques of Shiatsu

The principle of vertical and continuous pressure may appear obvious to all Shiatsu practitioners, but there are many other technical movements. Shiatsu is at the crossroads between massage, in the most traditional sense of the term, and Chinese acupressure. Moreover, we can trace the roots of this Japanese art back to ancient China (to at least 3000 years ago) to the name of Anmo Tuina. This term literally means "press" 按 (An), "rub" 摩 (Mó), "push" 推 (Tuī) and "grasp" 拿 (Ná). This technique, which is an integral part of Chinese medicine, historically gave Anma to Japan. During the Tokugawa period (Edo era), medical Anma (Kōhō Anma) was highly regarded and renowned. But a shogunal edict required that the blind should also be able to study Anma. This gave birth to the famous Anma san, people who played flutes in the streets to call customers. Little by little the medical Anma decreased, particularly from lack of literature, while the Anma of the blind became more and more popular. From the second half of the 19th to the beginning of the 20th century, some people sought to restore brilliance to the medical approach, which ultimately gave birth to Shiatsu.[1] The latter was adopted and recognized by the Japanese authorities, thanks to the public and political action of Tokujiro Namikoshi. The original Anma technique covered a wide range of technical movements. Some of these techniques are still found nowadays to a greater or lesser extent, depending on the style of Shiatsu practised.

Digitopressure

Shiatsu 指圧

Clearly, as we have seen before, vertical and continuous pressure is the basis of Shiatsu. But its purpose is not to randomly press on the body hoping to obtain a salutary effect. The pressure is mainly on the *tsubos* or Chinese meridian points. It is therefore necessary to be able not only to locate them, to feel them, but also to know their therapeutic effects. In addition to perpendicular pressure, other ways of touching points exist, as we shall see in the second part of this book. There is one notable exception to the precision of the points: Namikoshi's Shiatsu. While most practitioners are well trained in meridians, they proceed differently and choose to grid an anatomical area with several lines of points that are not necessarily related to the meridians, but more related to the musculature or tendons and ligaments. In this case the objective is not the same, but the results are relatively comparable.

Stretching

Jūnan taisō 柔軟体操

What would Shiatsu be without stretching? These movements consist of gently and deeply towing a part of the body, such as the four limbs, but also the neck, the spine, the sacrum, the ribs, etc. Stretching lengthens muscles and tendons, opens joints, and flushes toxins and lactic acid, a bit like wringing out a muscle as if it is a wet cloth. In addition, if maintained for a long time, it gently disconnects the sympathetic nervous system. The stretch always works from the surface of the muscle to its centre. So, we must not go too fast if we want to touch the depth and allow a real relaxation of body and mind. Each style of Shiatsu has its own way of performing stretching, but the common point is respect for anatomy. No one stretches an arm in a direction that is contrary to it and could hurt it. As a student, do not neglect to precisely study the art and the way of performing a good stretch without using force but by using the weight of the body, in order to maintain it as long as you want to.

Mobilizations

Kansetsu no kadō-sei 関節の可動性

A body with rusty joints is no longer functional and generates pain in movement. This is why mobilizations are part of the basic movements in the study of Shiatsu. The vast majority of recipients come to Shiatsu because they have pain in a muscle or joint. It is therefore essential to know how all the joints of the body work so as not to mistreat them, but also to know how to open them, soften them, and mobilize them correctly. Think for a minute about the shoulder. The variety of possible movements with a shoulder is impressive. The variety of the mechanical problems it may encounter is just as important. It is therefore necessary to know all the mobilization movements that exist to restore its mobility, and all this without causing more pain for the recipient. The study of mobilizations it therefore not a simple study, but is unfortunately often done too fast. In addition, the study of anatomy is essential to do a good job. Blocked joints tend to slow blood flow, block body fluids and stiffen due to an increase of collagen fibres. This leads to all kinds of complications such as stagnation of the blood, oedemas, concentration of toxins and various aches and pains. Be careful that the joint problem you are dealing with is within your field of expertise. Otherwise, rely on the help of a physiotherapist, an osteopath or even, in the most serious cases, the help of a doctor.

Friction

Keisatsu hō 軽擦法

Less known to students is that Shiatsu covers all kinds of friction of the body's tissues. This technique stimulates the skin, blood capillaries and nerve endings, and revives the so-called defensive Yang energy (*Wèi qì*) that is on the surface of the body. In the Chinese meridian system, friction is beneficial to re-energize the tiny communication meridians (the surface *Luò*), which in turn will stimulate the main meridians and their associated meridians (by Yin/Yang pair). Even though it is not the most common technique in Shiatsu, knowing how to use it wisely allows you to play with rhythms. To boost the energy of a recipient, it is a great technique to end a session in a tonic and pleasant way. To chase away depression, it is also recommended to rub the ribs for a long time. In short, friction has many virtues. In Chinese medicine, Anmo Tuina massage includes rubbing. But there is also another technique a little less known, *Guāshā* 刮痧 (literally "scratching cholera"), which involves scratching the skin using a curved stick, a smooth stone or a coin to chase the evil energy to the surface.

Kneading

Jūtetsu hō 柔てつ法

Purists will say that this is not part of Shiatsu because it is no longer perpendicular pressure. However, as with other technical movements, kneading muscles is very useful for relaxing tense areas. Working with the full palm or even with the fist is particularly practical in this case. Think of the back or glutes when they are hard. These are large muscles on which digitopressure will take a long time to act to obtain a correct relaxation. In addition, you are seriously at risk of hurting your fingers, especially your thumbs, if you do not go knead beforehand. You will gain in comfort of practice and relieve the joints of your fingers. Believing that Shiatsu is only digitopressure is a misunderstanding. Many styles of Shiatsu offer the use of massage techniques. This is why Shiatsu is commonly accepted by the public as a massage rather than an energetic and therapeutic technique. In reality, Shiatsu is often a mixture of both. Only putting pressure on *tsubos* is boring in the long run and makes us fall into the field of acupressure, which is a form of digital acupuncture.

Percussions

Dashin hō 打診法

There are many percussions in Shiatsu. Historically, they are a legacy from Anma massage. They have been upheld for their effectiveness and for being excellent at stimulating *Ki*. You can strike with the fists, the back of the hand, the two hands in a well shape or in a half-moon shape, etc.; there is no lack of techniques. It is quite amazing, for example, to receive 30 minutes of percussion on all or only part of the body within a Shiatsu. After a formal "bludgeoning", the recipient is always amazed by how much their muscles and nervous system have relaxed. In addition, just like friction, this strongly stimulates the circulation of energy, and a sensation of being in top form seems to appear out of nowhere. Athletes, actors and dancers are particularly fond of percussion, especially in preparation before a big event. The difference with friction is of course in the power and depth of the feeling. The practitioner must have a good amount of energy to do percussions for a long time. Without encouraging you to play the African drums, it is useful to have good health and a sense of rhythm to succeed in this technique. Hence the importance of maintaining yourself physically to keep good muscle tone.

Rocking

Kenbiki 腱引き

Rocking is as old as time. Indeed, it automatically reminds the body of the sway it experienced during its gestation in the mother's womb or in the arms of its parents at the beginning of its earthly life. Therefore, rocking is very effective for putting the sympathetic nervous system to sleep and triggering the parasympathetic, and also for putting the recipient in a state of primary well-being related to early childhood. It is also a very good technical movement to relax the muscles. Most muscles are organized longitudinally (on a Heaven–Earth axis) while most rocking is from right to left. Consequently, this puts the muscles in a different axis from the one in which they usually work, which allows them to let go relatively quickly. Thai massage uses a lot of rocking and Korean relaxation is entirely based on this principle. In Shiatsu, rocking is also used for relaxation and at the same time for diagnosis. If you shake an arm or leg, you learn a lot about muscle tension, joint flexibility, and the recipient's ability to stop wanting to control everything.

Vibrations

Shindō hō 振動法

This technical movement is not the most used or appreciated by practitioners, because it is difficult to achieve and quickly tiring. Yet it can be found in several schools as an integral part of the curriculum, because it makes sense. Vibrations send many tremors from the surface to the depth.[2] These vibrations help to stimulate the autonomic nervous system, but also to circulate stasis. For example, when the intestines are blocked, it can be painful to press on them. Well-placed vibrations will gently help to soften the knot causing the blockage.

Connections

Ki no rendō 気の連動

Connections are a good way to achieve energy circulation between two points or two hands. The basic principle is simple, but this subject deserves its own book as there is so much to say. Your two hands represent two poles of the same current. When you place them on the recipient's body, the energy they release will seek to connect, even if it is through another person. Once contact is established, a current is created and then strengthened, giving a pleasant feeling of warmth and re-energization. There are several ways to proceed in what some call fluidic Shiatsu.

- **Without intention**: simply place your hands in strategic places and let it flow, be calm and with presence.
- **With intention**: choose a path to travel, an organ to reach, an effect to trigger. This intention induces the path of energy or its effect. With a little training, it is even possible to choose the shape or movement to give energy from the transmitting hand.

In any case, the technique of connections is not done randomly. To succeed, it requires that all the basic prerequisites seen in the previous chapters are already in place. Then, it is necessary to know the reflex zones or the points, and the rules of associations between points to optimize the desired effect. Finally, we must be aware of what energy we release, day after day, so as not to burden the recipient with our undesirable aspects, nor risk exhaustion. This requires a self-awareness that is not within the reach of all beginners. This is why the technique of connections, even if it is simple to achieve and is within anyone's reach, is often considered an advanced aspect of Shiatsu.

All the techniques discussed in this chapter form the complex mixture that is Shiatsu. What often marks the personal style of one or the other practitioner is in the ways and means of mixing them, in the proportion he gives to one or the other technique, while managing to make everything fluid and harmonious.

Summary

1. There are many techniques within Shiatsu: perpendicular pressure, stretching, mobilization, vibration, percussion, friction, rocking, kneading and energetic connections.
2. This richness explains well what Shiatsu is: both a massage, digitopressure and an energy technique for therapeutic purposes.

12

Sensing

In a dream I shall feel its coolness on my feet.
I shall let the wind bathe my bare head.
I shall not speak, I shall think about nothing:
But endless love will mount in my soul;

EXCERPT FROM *SENSATION*, BY ARTHUR RIMBAUD[1]

An experienced practitioner can feel many sensations by simply touching the recipient. Better yet, he often manages to "pull up" information not only on the body, but also on the psychology and life of the person. For the neophyte this seems to be a kind of magic, although in reality the practitioner masters many ways of reading the body learned over the years. But, how do high-level practitioners know in a few minutes what is happening in a person? From habit certainly, but the habit of what exactly? How does this sensing work?

Sensing what?

First of all, each *shiatsushi* apprentice discovers that the main technical information is at their fingertips via palpation. This seemingly simple aspect alone requires several years of practice to mature. Whether you touch an organ, a muscle or an acupressure point, the basic information that the practitioner is looking for is always the same:

- **Kyo or jitsu**: is the affected area empty or hard, hollow, or too full?
- **Hot or cold**: does the affected area give a feeling of heat or cold?
- **Tonicity and elasticity**: does the affected area react quickly, does it return to its place as soon as it is let go or not? Is the flesh supple or taut or flaccid? In other words, we are looking for a healthy, flexible and yet firm point, otherwise it is not correct.

It is then possible to pass all this information through the mill of the Yin/Yang theories, the Five Movements and the eight therapeutic principles to begin to understand the logic of what is happening inside the person and to begin to formulate a coherent treatment. I put emphasis on the word "begin" because this step is just the start.

The study of palpation is progressive. It goes from studying the palpation of the back to that of the belly, through the meridians, points and pulses.

The study of pulses is relatively complex, especially if one wishes to master the 26 forms of Chinese pulse. Of course, it is not essential to know them all, but it is an excellent exercise to develop your sense of listening with your fingers. The more we practise palpation of the body, the more we improve our sensing. But for it to feel satisfying, you need:

- **Practice time**: the time factor is essential, because on one hand it increases the number of sensitive sensors (corpuscles of Pacini, Mesmer, Merkel, etc.) on the finger's surface and, on the other hand, because the experience fills and enriches your personal catalogue of sensations in order to establish links with the theory. This is one of the reasons why the study-time is long. We also know, especially through technical and neurological studies carried out on athletes and musicians, that it is necessary to spend at least 10,000 hours doing the same thing before you can be really good and effective in any field.[2] Shiatsu is no exception to the rule.
- **Calm**: without physical and mental calm, it is impossible to feel anything. This is why the regular practice of meditation is

the fastest way to learn to listen and hear what is not audible with the ear. As long as the mind is talkative, it is a distraction. In this case it will be impossible to capture other information than our own.

- **Letting go**: it is not enough to be calm, you must accept knowing nothing, controlling nothing and deciding nothing, regardless of your experience and the number of years of study. The practitioner does not control anything. He is available to the *jusha* and adapts to what he senses. Here we could take up the three basic rules of meditation that teach "do not force, do not seek and do not want". Through mental calmness and letting go, our body-mind whispers to us the most subtle information that we call "intuition". The practitioner can then bring out secrets buried in the recipient, who is not necessarily aware of them. Therefore, it is not magic, but listening and non-interference of one's own mind with the complex information system that is the human body.

Finding the elusive

There are many exercises to develop your senses, and each school will be keen to develop its own. Among the educational games that can be designed to develop sensing in students, the most obvious and easiest to do is to work after a good warm-up and a meditation session. The body and mind then become more receptive than normal.

Another fun and educational exercise is to blindfold a student using a *tenugi* or any scarf. He will then be asked to palpate the body and describe the muscles, or to do a massage, or to follow a meridian. This is a good exercise for memorizing the paths of the meridians but also a great way to develop the sense of touch for more advanced students. I recommend doing this for students who are trying their hand at diagnosis by palpation. Depriving ourselves of sight, our most used sense, allows us to focus on others (smell, hearing and, of course, touch). During intensive courses, you can do a variant by performing Shiatsu at night, without turning on the lights of course.

The human body is usually cluttered with all sorts of toxins that literally clog the digestive system. By changing our eating pattern, especially by lightening it, the body becomes lighter and intestinal transit more fluid. Our intestines include what is called the second brain,[3] with 530 million neurons. By improving intestinal transit, these neurons can function optimally. The belly starts to "think" less about itself and becomes more available for feeling. What is called instinct comes directly from "the gut". By lightening it and caring for it, you make it more effective, and your instincts will become sharper and sharper. Practising Shiatsu in a period of fasting is also a quite an amazing experience because of the power and clarity of feeling it brings.

If you think of sensing like the *bunshin* phase[4] of the diagnosis, it is said that you have to feel the recipient. This can be understood in two different ways. Sensing means feeling the sensations but could also mean using olfaction.[5] Ohashi Sensei is probably the most surprising master in this field. He can detect a sick person and sometimes identify the disease just by passing by, using only his sense of smell. According to him, the "trick" to smelling correctly is to radically change your diet to modify your body odour. Thus, by modifying his odour compared to others, it is possible to better smell that of others. But if you eat like them, it remains difficult or impossible.

In Shiatsu, it is not necessary to do long studies to realize that two human bodies harmonize after a few minutes of contact. Anyone, even uninitiated in Shiatsu, can experience it. This harmonization will gain speed and depth with years of experience. An experienced practitioner will be able to place his hand on a recipient and their bodies will harmonize their breathing and energies within less than a minute. Thanks to this, exchanges happen easily between the two bodies, without a single word being spoken. The practitioner will then extend his energy beyond his own hands to enter the recipient's body. Thanks to inner calm and this depth of action, the information will naturally come to him. For the rest, he must trust himself and accept the images, thoughts, words and even songs or tunes that come to him spontaneously. Professor Stéphane Vien describes sessions where suddenly a chorus of a song comes to him, such as *I will survive*, without knowing that his client has been fighting for a long time against a serious illness. Everything is information. My advice is to accept all this but to remain cautious and keep this information to yourself, to use it only to cross-check your diagnosis without sinking into superfluous interpretations, at the risk of being mistaken. Know how to remain humble.

Feeling the energy

What student has never declared that he is no good because he can't feel the energy! This is quite normal because to feel *Ki*, you have to go through a whole education of the body and listening. The first obstacle that prevents us from feeling energy is the idea that we have of it. Too often popular culture reminds us of *Star Wars* and the Jedi, or electricity and lightning. These mental projections must disappear before you can feel *Ki*. Once calm is present, any beginner will know how to feel a current, a crackle. When I teach, I can quickly guide students on the feeling of energy passing through their fingers, usually at the end of the first year. The first time that this happened to me, I had six years of study behind me, and I was in despair. Then one evening, it happened and was so strong and beautiful that the tears began to flow by themselves. Obviously, the next day when I wanted to repeat the experience, nothing came and it took me six more months to systematize this feeling, so patience. Good things come to those who wait and remain self-confident. I will quote Henri-Frédéric Amiel:[6] "Happiness is made of energy, perseverance and faith: if you want to attract it to you, without tiring, work and pray." On the other hand, knowing how to detect variations in this current requires a few more years of practice, proof that there is always more to learn and that's good!

Energy is a natural phenomenon that, according to scientists, is produced by the body and circulates in it. This is called bioenergy. For the ancient Chinese, it is a larger phenomenon found at all levels in the universe, nature and living beings, which circulates and gives life to all things. We will further explore the notion of energy in Chapter 16 among the advanced concepts of Shiatsu.

Summary

1. The basic feeling concerns: *kyo* or *jitsu*, hot or cold, tonic or flaccid?
2. Develop the sense of touch, especially by avoiding the use of sight.
3. Developing sensing allows you to capture subtle information coming from the receiver.
4. To get a good feeling, it takes time, calm and letting go.
5. The feeling of energy (Qì) is possible, and even beginners can do it. But identifying variations in Qì requires years of regular practice.

13

Without Force

What a divine artist, as to the ancient wrestler,
Gave you so much strength with so much beauty?

EXCERPT FROM *POEME TO ALFRED DE MUSSET*, BY FÉLIX ARVER[1]

The strength described in the short excerpt above reminds us of Greek marble statues whose every muscle is drawn to perfection. We can see here all the strength of a Hercules or an Achilles, but these are images where the force is retained inside, contained in the white stone. This strength does not need to exert itself to get a result and impress us. This is exactly what we ask of Shiatsu students and practitioners. Not using arm strength is probably what gives Shiatsu students the most trouble, except perhaps those who practise martial arts... and only perhaps! Yet one might think that doing nothing is very simple. In reality, nothing is more complicated than implementing simplicity. The reason for the difficulty of work without strength lies in our education.

All our lives we have been told that we must make efforts, push with all our strength, be the first, run faster and not relax in terms of effort. Not to mention that you don't get anything without effort. Starting with such assumptions, it is not surprising to see students struggling not to use strength. All our education is oriented towards doing – do more, do better, do not sit idly by and do nothing, do it and do it again and again until you succeed. The Western mind is entangled in the idea that the result comes at the end of efforts and that it is necessary to work tirelessly until a hypothetical success is achieved. If we add to this the capitalist myth of success at all costs, whatever the cost, we understand better that success without additional means is not in our capacity for immediate understanding. Who in your life, parent or teacher, has ever told you to sit down, not move, breathe and focus on not-doing and not-thinking? On the contrary, the Taoist mind is entirely turned towards non-action: *Wú wéi* (無爲). The world is well organized enough to run without us and brings to everyone what they need. "The wise man does not act" said the *Dao De Jing*.[2]

Removing muscle strength

Do nothing yes, but not just anyhow. Using a technique without strength requires a good understanding of postures, especially with movement. If the posture is correct, the *shiatsushi*'s body does not strain and does not hurt. Therefore, he does not need to contract involuntarily to compensate for his posture failings. From here, he will always be well placed in relation to the body of the receiver; this will avoid having to use strength or move. This placing will allow him to be permanently above the area to be pressured. All he has to do is shift his centre of gravity and let the weight of his body create pressure.

Technically speaking, to succeed in not putting strength in the movement, it is not necessary to:

- use the shoulder muscles
- use the muscles of the arms and extend the elbows
- use the muscles of the hands and fingers.

In short, no muscular strength should be applied from the shoulders and fingertips to succeed in Shiatsu pressure. It is obviously tempting to do the opposite (especially unconsciously). Beginners often say that they believe they are doing well by adding strength. Not only is it useless, but by adding strength to the pressure you run the risk of:

- not feeling the limit when the pressure is no longer tolerated by the receiver
- hurting the receiver, which will put you into failure
- wearing out your cartilage and therefore being in pain in the long run.

On the contrary, by suppressing muscle strength and using only the movement of your weight from the hips, you cannot push beyond the resistance of the recipient's body. This way, you never risk hurting them, while retaining enough potential to gently enter the tissues. Your pressure will always be adapted to their ability to receive, respecting the sensitivity of the receiver which is thus preserved. In addition, you will not wear out your joints, which are particularly fragile in the wrists and fingers, which is not unimportant. In short, as we are used to saying, *less is more*.[3] This postulate can be formulated in a more amusing way: "The law of the laziest is always the best." At least for the practice of Shiatsu.

Women, who do not have as much muscle as men, know very early on in life that they will not be able to rely on the strength of their arms alone to get out of various situations. They then rely on their sensitivity, reasoning and body movement. Being generally more focused on their belly than men (for obvious anatomical reasons), they quickly do wonders in Shiatsu and are capable of releasing a great and soft power. To understand this, one must clearly make the distinction between strength and power.

Difference between strength and power

Strength is the result of muscular action. Imagine that you must push someone heavier than you. Using your muscles may hurt them, but certainly not move them. Why? Because by using your muscle strength, you are not using anything like your full potential, only a part of it (mostly arms or legs). As soon as the whole body moves, it also moves a mass, which means a weight and a volume. By combining strength and movement of the body, you set power in motion. The more the movement starts from the centre of the body, the deeper the power that is expressed and the more impossible it is to counter. Discovering how to increase the power of the body is at the heart of all martial systems.

Shiatsu used power without strength, without aggressiveness, and therefore without capacity to do harm. These are exactly the same principles as those used for Aikidō, martial art that is unique because it does not seek performance and refuses competition. For those who seek how to put a person on the ground without using force or violence, I can only recommend that they explore this complementary path. Moreover, for passionate researchers, I recommend following the triple path of meditation, Shiatsu and martial arts, which are three different forms exploiting the same principles. Their studies reinforce each other exponentially.

Benefits of working without force

By mobilizing the power of the body, the *shiatsushi* is able to achieve a deep yet painless action on the body of the recipient, an important but not traumatic pressure, a penetration of the flesh that is never intrusive. Better still, this work without strength makes it possible to install a beautiful presence for the practitioner who nevertheless leaves room for the recipient to feel himself without suffering a constraint or an authoritarian point of view. Work without strength is the keystone of technical success in Shiatsu. The presence of pain would not allow the recipient to:

- let go physically and even less mentally
- find a framework of trust that he is entitled to expect by going to a professional
- release physical tension or drop emotional baggage
- recover by activating the parasympathetic nervous system.

This last point is fundamental. In Shiatsu we talk about prompting the self-healing forces that lie dormant in any individual, in order to repair internal imbalances and harmonize the body and its energies. Harmonizing when pain occurs is simply impossible.[4] In addition, aiming to improve physical and energetical condition is just as important, because it is the parasympathetic system that cleanses the body, repairs it, re-energizes it as it regulates vegetative functions. As long as pain is present, the brain will not let go and the sympathetic nervous system will remain in control. Problem: this nervous system does not know how to repair the body, quite the contrary. It participates in the catabolism of the body, in the deconstruction of its molecular components in order to release energy. The parasympathetic nervous system participates in the anabolic cycle that recomposes the body by molecular synthesis. We can see here the whole point of working without strength to guide the receiver in a physical and mental area where he will give himself the means to repair himself.

Bypassing the blockage

Another not insignificant advantage of working without strength is the possibility of overcoming painful blockages. As has been said, the movement of the practitioner's body from the centre, and without arm strength, makes it possible to fall right into a tension, a knot, a contracture, without risking exceeding the threshold of tolerance to pain of the recipient. That's good, but it's just the beginning. If you really want to do a treatment in the sense of "relieving the person", you need to go further and overcome the blockage. Pay attention to this nuance: relieving pain and relieving a person is not the same intention and does not require the same work. Yet one is the first step on the other's path. So, let's get back to that first step. To relieve pain, several options are available to you:

- Wait on the painful spot, always without forcing, until it softens, opens and relaxes completely. It may take more or less time, but it is a risk-free approach.
- Create a movement of energy dispersion on the knot, in particular by turning counterclockwise. Indeed, a tension knot requires a high concentration of energy in a very localized point. Scatter the energy and the knot will slowly unravel after a while. It can also take more or less time.
- The Sei Shiatsu of Bernard Bouheret offers an unusual technique which consists of sucking up the contacted tension, then releasing even more the body of the *shiatsushi*. This technique must be studied because it involves a subtle understanding of breathing and body management. Its advantage is immense because the result is almost immediate, and in just a few seconds we can feel the thumbs passing beyond the resistance of the tissues.

Remember that these techniques are only possible because at the basis of the movement there was no strength in the arms, nor intention to fight against resistance, but a benevolent and irresistible power. It is therefore essential to learn to let go of the desire to succeed, to force the passage, to have a result at all costs. The best advice we can give here is to accept that the technique is self-sufficient. You have to trust it and yourself. And above all, relax.

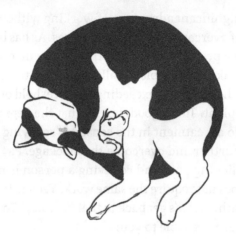

One day a 40-year-old man, manager of a gymnastics club, came for a problem of mental or professional overload; he did not know which, except that he could not take any more. Yet his body, as his job requires, was of impeccable tone and musculature and one would have thought that he could endure anything. But all living beings have their limit, and this was expressed by terrible stomach-aches that hit him from time to time, at any time of the day, which is a considerable handicap. I could feel a hard belly and decided to work on the rest of the body rather than the belly. The person, astonished, asked me why I was dodging his problem which was obviously in the belly. I replied that I was working like him, that I was dodging the problem that led him to have a stomach-ache. He went through several emotions, became white, then red. Once he turned pink again and his breathing calmed down, I asked him if he was now ready to get to the heart of the problem. After his agreement, I placed my fingers on the points of the Spleen called "the knot of the belly" (Sp 14) and "the complaint of the belly" (Sp 16). He moaned in pain for at least a minute or two, blowing like a whale. Then the tensions dissipated, his intestines made loud noises and he had to hastily empty himself on the toilet of stool which he described to me as "acidic" and "burning". That same evening, he had a heated but essential discussion with his wife, telling her that he loved her but that he could no longer accept being psychologically abused. He never had a stomach-ache again, but taken by a passion for Shiatsu, he became a student the following school year. This is the beauty of Shiatsu: by liberating men and women, you allow them to transform.

Summary

1. Working without strength always allows you to get the right pressure.
2. It offers the patient a reassuring and non-restrictive feeling.
3. It prevents the *shiatsushi* from getting tired and wearing out his joints.
4. It helps to understand the difference between strength and power.
5. It provides the means to overcome the blockages of body and mind.

Man

Advanced Principles
and Concepts

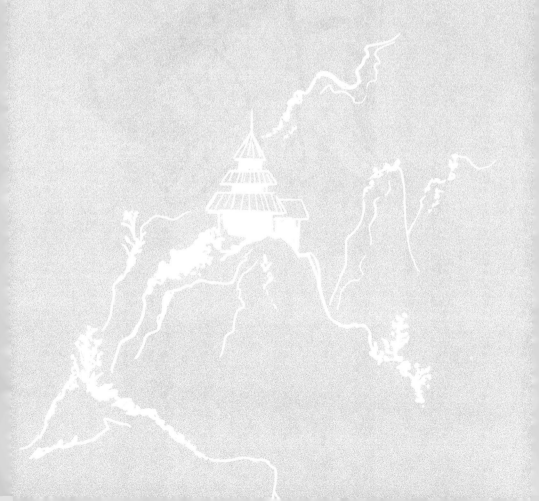

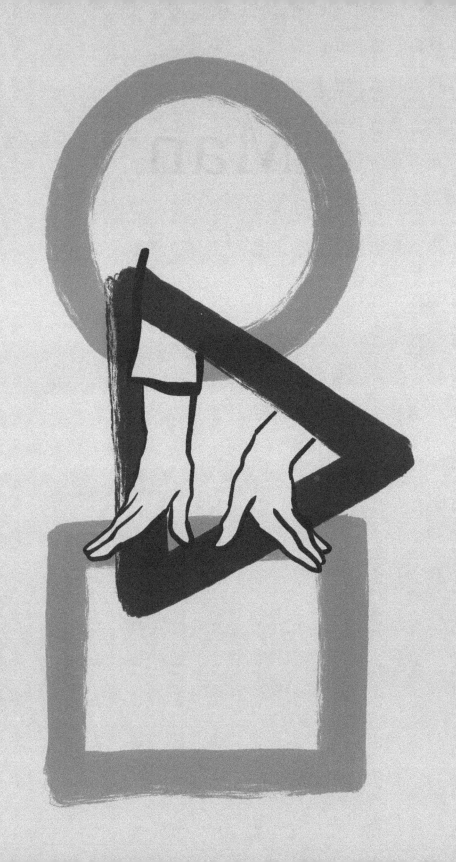

Explanation of
Advanced Principles

To understand the concepts that make up the advanced principles of our discipline, let's remember what Shiatsu is: a *Do*, a Way. To deny this fact or to reduce Shiatsu to a simple mechanical technique is like missing out on a treasure that is being handed to you with both hands. In Japan, China and the Far East in general it is understood that trades and arts are not simply techniques. Rather, they are a way to individual fulfilment, ways of growing beyond the gestures and theories. A Way serves to transcend technique and to fulfil oneself as a human being. From the point of view of Shiatsu, this is to be in harmony with nature in general and with our human nature in particular, taking responsibility for the environment, and to recognize and live nature within oneself, following its cycles and needs. It also means accepting our responsibilities as a human being to our fellow human beings, and accepting the burden, the role and the efforts required to become a genuine therapist.

It's a whole programme, an individual journey that sometimes takes many detours and inevitably many years.

To grasp the advanced principles of Shiatsu, we must inevitably go through meditation, in both senses of the word–the Western sense, where we think deeply about a subject, and the Eastern sense, where we seek to reach a state without thought. And so, little by little, the Shiatsu practitioner not only gains in knowledge and understanding thanks to his readings and reflections, but he also gains in calm, in feeling, in clarity of mind and in intuition, in short, into the depths of his practice. Through meditation – in the broadest sense of the term – he conceptualizes more advanced principles, even if they are similar in appearance to the basic principles.

In the first part of this book, the basic principles were concrete, mechanical, and fairly easy to implement. Go to a good school and in just three or four years you will have mastered them more or less correctly. The advanced principles, on the other hand, reveal a more inner, subtle and demanding dimension. The steps follow each other, each principle flows directly from the application of the previous one. I have tried to classify them – as far as possible, because Eastern thought is not linear – in the following logical order to help you understand them better. But this way of explaining things is by no means an absolute truth, just the fruit of my experience.

These principles offer practitioners the means to progress through life and touch the depths of Shiatsu. Martial arts practitioners will not be confused by the terms used here, as they are often the same as those used in Japanese disciplines. And this is quite normal, as all the Ways are guided by the same principles, whatever technique used and whatever society we come from.

14

Cleansing and Purification

Fly far, far away from this baneful miasma
And purify yourself in the celestial air,
Drink the ethereal fire of those limpid regions
As you would the purest of heavenly nectars.

EXCERPT FROM *ELEVATION*, BY CHARLES BAUDELAIRE[1]

The first part of this book deliberately does not discuss the warm-up and preparation of the body as basic principles essential to a good Shiatsu. This would have reduced the practitioner's preparation to a simple body technique when it is not. In the Far Eastern mind, body and mind are one.[2] This is why it is inconceivable that a warm-up or preparation is only physical, unless there is really a lack of time, but this must be the exception rather than the rule. In addition, preparing the body like an athlete would really be the minimum service that a Shiatsu practitioner can give to his client. More than a musculo-articular preparation, the practitioner must work his body and mind to cleanse them of their *kegare* 穢れ (dregs) to clarify the inside. This is the meaning of the word *misogi* (禊) which means "cleansing" or "purification" in Japanese.

Cleanse and purify

This notion is found in martial arts where the cleansing of the body is the basis of training. Originally, the practice of *misogi* comes from the Shintō religion (神道). It is a meditation that is practised under a waterfall so that it cleanses the body and mind. This is practised at any time of the year, but there are two more intense *misogi*, one at the coldest of winter and the other at the hottest of summer. The idea is to go beyond one's resistance and one's usual physical and mental capacities to rediscover oneself, to go beyond one's limits by letting go deep within oneself. On a daily basis, *misogi* is less intense, but it is a ritual that brings the Shiatsu practitioner back to this personal quest for improvement. By the way, this quest for improvement is also a principle called *Kaizen* (改善).

A master like Masanori Okamoto of Kuretake Shiatsu is used to pouring a bucket of cold water on his body, regardless of the season. Takeuchi Sensei of Yin Shiatsu also practised it for years. This is why this cleansing is conceived as "chasing the slag" from the body. If for example in the morning you do the *makōhō* 真向法 (stretching of the meridians), you seek to cleanse the energy channels of the body to fluidify the flow of *Ki* through them. While visibly stretching the muscles, you scan the channels with your mind to keep everything clean and functional. Cleaning your practice area every morning is part of the same idea. *Misogi* is also found in the forging of metal. For the warrior's sword to be resistant, it must be purified of all the slag of the ore in order to obtain the purest metal and therefore the hardest.

This notion of cleansing then engages the individual in a process of purification, which is called *harai* (祓) in Japanese. As incarnate beings, we can never be 100 per cent completely pure. By definition, humans have strengths but also weaknesses, they are not absolute. On the other hand, one can tend towards this absolute and make efforts towards it. In the context of Shiatsu, this daily purification is of great importance. If we take the example of *makōhō*, you clean the meridians of their blockages. But let's imagine that you feel a sharper pain than usual in the meridians of the Spleen and Liver. You remember then that you exaggerated last night during a drunken evening with good friends. You will not try to dodge this pain by taking pain medications, but rather dive into your sensations, purge the affected meridians and purify your mind of the reason that pushed you to drink so much, just so you don't start again any time soon.

Misogi and *harai* are two concepts that work together; one has no meaning without the other. For example, meditation is a good tool to purify one's mind of all our thoughts, but without work on the body, it has much less scope. The reverse is also true. This is why meditation under a waterfall is a test for the mind (strengthening one's will) and for the body (resisting water pressure and cold). There are many forms of *misogi harai*, almost as many as there are arts and techniques. In Aikidō, Nobuyoshi Tamura Sensei used a system from Shiatsu, a kind of mixture of auto-Shiatsu by pressing certain points and *makōhō*. That being said, Aikidō itself includes *misogi harai* exercises more related to Shintō rituals such as repeating the same technique 500 or 1000 times in a row. This is the case of *suburi* 素振 (cutting in the void with a wooden sword) or *ukemi* 受け身 (falling on the tatami). The body cannot do this exercise without exhausting itself quickly and the mind demands that all this stop as quickly as possible.

I experienced these exercises when I was an Aikidō student.[3] My teacher would push us until we fainted or vomited. Despite this, we had to come back, continue, hold on. To succeed in these exercises, you must let go of your immediate little desires, your pain and even the idea of doing the exercise. The mind (re)discovers itself firmer and more voluntary than it could imagine itself. Nakazono Sensei,[4] another great master of Aikidō and Shiatsu, regularly performed a sequence of 50 dynamic postures.[5] Yoga can be considered as a *misogi harai* as one immediately feels the benefits at the end of a session, the feeling of being more flexible, longer and cleaner inside. Many Shiatsu teachers also use Tàijíquán or Qìgōng. These two arts, often confused, cleanse the body and purify the mind to access a dimension without desire, just for the pleasure of living and feeling an empty mind in a full body.

Cleansing exercises

Martial arts are not the only ones to use the concepts of *misogi harai*. There are also many Shiatsu exercises that meet this need to cleanse and purify the practitioner. Not only does *misogi harai* strengthen the mind, but it cleanses the body so well that it prevents it from getting sick, which is a good example when one claims to want to balance people and keep them healthy. To purify the Liver meridian, Kawada Sensei likes to do the splits, cross his arms and then swing vigorously from right to left a good hundred times. Or to strengthen the will, he puts himself in *kibadachi* 騎馬立ち (iron rider position) and holds out until all his students have collapsed on the ground, which can take quite a long time. In another style, Ohashi Sensei rubs all over his body to activate the skin and increase the circulation of surface energy. Kobayashi Sensei, the oldest teacher at the Japan Shiatsu College in Tokyo, scrupulously assesses all the joints of his body and works them until they are all flexible and without a glitch. It is surprising to see this man of more than 70 years old leave everyone breathless when he walks, supple and fast. For my part, during the winter I like to perform a *kata* of 17 movements specifically for the Ki of the Kidneys, which warms the body and raises the energy potential so strongly that it is not advisable to do it too often.

Misogi harai can also come into a wide variety of practices because, between body and mind, it is of course possible to emphasize one or the other. Meditation consists of letting the energy of breath flow freely in the body and emptying one's mind. But through meditation it is also possible to evoke images to purify oneself, such as dropping a celestial light on oneself, like a shower that cleans/purifies every cell of the body. There is also a meditative technique called *Chinkon kishin*. The translation is quite complex, something like "sinking into the soul" or "putting the soul in the body", or perhaps even "pacifying the soul". This includes specific hand postures, hand gestures and visualizations. It mainly plays on a breathing based on a rhythm of 7 seconds minimum: breathe in for 7 seconds, 7 seconds in apnea, and breathe out for 7 seconds.

From the first cycles, the mind calms down and very quickly it purifies itself of its thoughts.

Kototama (the art of using sounds) is a technique that cleanses energy. Each sound expressed by the mouth has a vibratory length. The simple use of vowels or certain consonants makes the body vibrate on one frequency or another. The simplest method is to hold a vowel as long as possible, in a loud and clear voice. Once you have sung a, e, i, o, u, start again by changing the octave, and so on until you can't any more, then suddenly be silent. You will feel the body vibrate on all levels, especially the chakras. As you now can understand, any way of doing *misogi harai* engages the body-mind. These exercises are to be given to students so that they can discover a wide range of tools that address both the coarse (muscles) and the subtle (energy), through the mind and finally the spirit.

Ongoing work

In the professional practice of Shiatsu, purification occurs throughout the day. In the morning to get started, to limber and warm up the body, *misogi harai* is often done dynamically. Between each appointment, washing your hands with soap and cold water is not only a hygienic gesture but also a purification that drains accumulated energies. At the end of the day, a soft and inner *misogi harai* (through the breath in particular) allows to find oneself after having given oneself generously. It especially cleanses the body of emotions and thoughts that are not necessarily those of the practitioner. Thus, we cut off from the different people we have touched, to avoid carrying their imbalances, mental slag and other pathological disorders. Japanese masters speak of inner polishing, of always working on oneself so that our inner substance shines like a mirror.

The warrior polishes his blade
Suddenly, a burst
Flight of larks[6]

Misogi harai is therefore not an intellectual stance to annoy young practitioners. It is a practice that is both an invigorating revitalization that gives strength, calm and flexibility, and a necessity so that the practitioner does not tire. This last notion is rarely mentioned in Shiatsu. Seen from the outside as a client or even as a student, one often gets the impression that the practitioner or teacher is always fit and seems indestructible. Nothing could be further from the truth. They are human beings like any other. In addition, the practice of Shiatsu can be physically, energetically and psychically exhausting. Mobilizing heavy bodies, massaging hard muscles, relaxing stiff joints is already a challenge that requires good stamina. Feeling the energy, nourishing it, unlocking it, rebalancing it is a second job that needs a large reserve of energy and the ability to connect with Heaven and Earth to not be completely drained. Finally, accompanying the anguish and tears, listening to the pains and tragedies of humanity that parade through our hands requires great centring and immense inner strength. This is why the practice of *misogi harai* is to be done to allow a renewal and reinforcement of each day.

On the other hand, avoiding this personal work amounts to ensuring physical and psychological fatigue that can go as far as exhaustion and complete cessation of practice. We know that burn-out syndrome appeared in the hospital environment of the 1960s in the United States. Today, it affects almost all professions, but the most affected population is that of doctors and health practitioners in the broad sense. Burn-out is not just a great exhaustion of the energy of the body but also a void of spiritual energy (*Shén*). Using meditation, *misogi harai* and other techniques, the practitioner places his day and his Shiatsu practice on another, higher level. He does not repeat the same technique every day otherwise he would be deeply bored and, after several years, wearied. By placing one's daily practice at the spiritual level, Shiatsu and all the gestures that surround it take on a whole new meaning that nourishes and strengthens the individual and makes him grow internally. Thus, the practitioner begins to walk on what is called Shiatsu Dō (the Shiatsu Way). Doing *misogi harai* is therefore one of the fundamental aspects for a sustainable and in-depth practice of Shiatsu.

Summary

1. The practitioner follows a daily cleansing before, during and after a working day.
2. The work of cleansing makes it possible to tend towards the purification of one's mind.
3. Forgetting *misogi harai* will quickly weigh down the body and mind and tire the practitioner.
4. There are many exercises for *misogi harai*. The practitioner may vary these according to his needs for cleansing the body, mind or even energy.
5. *Misogi harai* places the daily practice of Shiatsu in another dimension than just technique. It spiritualizes the practitioner and strengthens his spirit.

15

Internal Strength

Previously, we saw that without correct posture Shiatsu simply does not exist, at least technically speaking. But the term "posture" has a double meaning. We will use the term to mean both how one physically positions oneself and also moral posture. The moral posture is the set of rules that a person applies to themselves in a given context, whether in society, their profession or for all the acts of their daily life. It dictates their behaviour towards themselves and others. Shiatsu being both a path of individual development and of relationship with others, moral posture is at the basis of our personal and professional ethics.

Strength in form

In Japanese, the word *Shisei* 姿勢 gives us valuable information on this aspect. The two kanji (Japanese ideograms) that compose it read as follows:

- *Sugata* (姿 pronounced *shi* in this case) expresses strength, appearance, size.
- *Ikioi* (勢 pronounced *sei*) expresses strength, what is correct, good, fair.

Therefore, *Shisei* reads "strength in the form" or "behaviour with vigour", which is more prosaically translated as posture or attitude. But not just any attitude: the correct, upright posture. Thanks to this correct posture, the individual can release a vigour, an inner strength that is immediately seen in its external manifestations: vitality, quality and power of movements, bright eyes, controlled strength, etc.

But the term *Shisei* is not limited to having a well-balanced body, straight back and arms in the axis of the hips. It also requires relaxation and centring. If you adopt a correct position but you are on guard, chest swollen forward and back stiff, you will get tired, that's for sure. In addition, *Ki* will not flow properly if there are tensions of all kinds between different parts of the body. For this, drop the shoulders and breathe into the belly (*hara*). With the help of breathing – and with a little practice – the body gently undulates on its front line as well as on its back line (spine). This is exactly what happens in the *seiza* 正座 ("correct sitting") position that is used in everyday life in Japan. Everything is straight but nothing is fixed. In this way, we understand once again the intimate relationship that exists between Shiatsu and meditation. To have *Shisei* is to put in order the body, this vessel that contains and develops *Ki*, to make it strong. And to make it strong, you must lower the breath into the belly and release all tension.

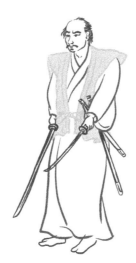

MIYAMOTO MUSASHI, INVENTOR OF THE SCHOOL OF
THE TWO SWORDS HYŌHŌ NITEN ICHI RYŪ.

The great swordsman Miyamoto Musashi[1] said, speaking of the martial *Shisei*:

The face is calm, neither turned upwards, nor downwards, nor to the side, the eyes slightly closed, without any movement of the eyeballs, the forehead without a fold, the eyebrows slightly furrowed, the ridge of the nose straight, without bringing the chin too far forward, the neck is also straight, the cervical vertebrae full of strength. Below the dropped shoulders, the body is perfectly relaxed, the spine is in place, the buttocks tucked in; from knees to toes pressed strongly on the floor, the hips are not twisted, the belly is firmly rounded.

Isn't this the exact description of posture in Shiatsu?

Benefits of katas

For the Asian mind, the best way to learn is to physically repeat a movement until the body integrates it without having to go through the intellect. The pedagogical principle boils down to doing rather than explaining. To do this, the Japanese invented the *kata* 型 ("mould, trace, ideal shape"), a sequence of movements that are repeated. The *kata* is shown little by little to the student, without explaining the ins and outs. When one movement is acquired, he learns the next, and so on until the end of the sequence. The equivalent Chinese term is *dàolù* (道路). It gives us a deeper meaning of what a sequence is because *dàolù* literally means "the path on the Way". What appears to be a simple succession of technical gestures is much more than that. It is a tool for knowledge and self-discovery.

A *kata* works like a chest of drawers. In the first drawer is the physical form, visible, external. It must be repeated over and over again to get the keys that open the second drawer. Each movement gives access to a key that leads to a deeper understanding. The visible technical movement leads to the invisible technical depth. This depth leads to technical efficiency. Technical efficiency leads to bodily and mental relaxation. This relaxation leads to energy circulation. Energy circulation opens the body–mind to a deeper and spontaneous understanding of technique. This depth gives access to the principles underlying the technique. The *kata* then takes on its full educational meaning and allows us to rediscover the purpose of the visible movements. It is a virtuous circle, which goes from the surface to the depth to rise to the surface and create an endless movement between the visible and the invisible.

Kata is not just a silly repetition. It is empty. I realize it now, the *kata* is like a huge library, without books, but which frees the body and the mind.[2]

Creating a *kata* is not an easy task; it is the result of a lifetime of study and teaching. Asian masters who created a martial or Shiatsu *kata* did so with the idea of allowing the student to move from one level of understanding to another, without using words. It's a body language. Westerners like to analyse, dissect and discuss the composition of a *kata*, but this is not useful. It must be repeated and repeated again to obtain the substantive marrow. It is the way of a lifetime. Knowing this, it is essential to follow the movements millimetre by millimetre. There is also no point in questioning the movements of a *kata*. This attitude shows that we are far from having understood all its depth and the hidden meanings that the master has distilled in the technique, layer by layer, level by level, for the elevation of the student able to work on it for decades. When there are several katas in a school, we usually realize that the first of them, the simplest, holds the most essential lessons.

Therefore, it is not for nothing that in Shiatsu many schools teach at least one *kata*. The best known is Tokujiro Namikoshi's *kata*, but there are many others. In Sei Shiatsu, Bernard Bouheret extensively teaches a *kata*, the fruit of more than 30 years of work. The Kōhō Shiatsu school is a martial school and proceeds in the same way. Other schools teach katas per season, per emotion or per Element. Each *kata* seeks to meet one need or another, but in any case, the *kata* offers a pedagogical framework to find and discover posture, relaxation, effectiveness, depth, and many other aspects of Shiatsu. As it is not possible to break from the visible form, it is gradually discovered that the *kata* forges a powerful and anchored body. Over the years, this body will develop another aspect of the practitioner's personality: his mental strength.

Shisei mind

By extrapolation, the word *Shisei* enlightens us about the moral attitude of the practitioner. He does not let himself be fooled by customer recriminations or congratulations. His ego no longer seeks the passing glory of successful treatment and the disappearance of symptoms. He seeks only to place himself at the service of his art by applying himself as best he can, with all his presence and inner strength. He agrees to let each person choose their path of healing. Even if he proposes and considers quick solutions that he knows well, he must not force the hand of the person who comes to meet him but let the person go at his own pace. And regardless of the number of years of study and the extent of his skills, the practitioner remains aware of not being a healer. He is the caregiver, the accompanist, the walking stick that supports the person on his inner journey, the mid-wife who allows awareness through feeling, the trigger of the living forces of self-healing. But he never holds the solution. He circulates the solution through him to allow each person to regain his balance, to resume his path of life and not to remain in the disease.

Sincerity

Thanks to his demeanour, the *Shisei* mind then changes into *Seishin* (正心). Both kanji mean "right, true" and "heart, mind". *Seishin* then takes on the meaning of the practitioner's moral righteousness, of his sincerity. The founder of Shiatsu, Tenpeki Tamai, dedicates an entire chapter of his book *Shiatsu hō* to *Seishin*.[3] He says: "a practitioner must have an advanced *Seishin* to accomplish the various methods discussed in this book":

- *Reite Shiatsu Ryōhō* 靈手指壓療法 ("Shiatsu Therapy by the Spirit of the Hand" or "by the Spiritual Hand")
- *Shiatsu Ryōhō Kanshinjutsu* 指壓療法觀心術 ("Art of contemplation in Shiatsu therapy")
- *Shiatsu Ryōhō Anjijutsu* 指壓療法暗示術 ("Art of suggestion in Shiatsu therapy")
- *Shiatsu Ryōhō Shinrigaku* 指壓療法心理學 ("Study of the state of mind in Shiatsu therapy").

As we can see, the spiritual aspect and the state of mind needed to perform Shiatsu were the main concerns of its founder.[4] Therefore,

Seishin represents the path of consistency and personal discipline, which opens access to the spiritual dimension of Shiatsu. At this level of understanding, the practitioner has assimilated the technical movements and digested the advanced concepts. He has put into practice his position between Earth and Heaven and agreed to be the connecting thread of the great forces of Yin/Yang. He moves from a horizontal position (earth to earth) to a vertical position by stretching his mind towards Heaven. It takes great moral strength and true physical and spiritual discipline to get to this stage. Then, the celestial *Ki* and terrestrial *Ki* will flow naturally thanks to this vertical stretching. *Shisei* then becomes the notion that allows you to pass from body to heart, from heart to mind and from mind to body. As Michel Odoul says very well in his book on the Japanese spirit,[5] "this triple work makes it possible to distinguish without difficulty the great practitioners from the vulgar". In this way, he carries on and internalizes his personal work in order to raise his mind and train his Heart (with a capital H) and his technique by pulling them upwards. It is the work of a lifetime that takes the status of Shiatsu from manual technique to a magnificent Way that fills a lifetime.

If we forget this ongoing quest for righteousness, *Seishin* and *Shisei* empty themselves of their strength, and in the long run the technique becomes repetitive, boring, the practitioner loses his inner strength. We keep the back straight (just about) to avoid pain, but it stops there. After a few years we no longer find meaning in what we do, and we have forgotten the urge transmitted to us by our masters and which motivated us so much when we were students. Unfortunately, I have had the opportunity to see the accuracy of these words in my life. A person who was studying Shiatsu at the same time as me finished his studies with enthusiasm. Then little by little, he began to mix the technique with other unrelated contributions, to question that required effort in Shiatsu, to criticize my desire to search; finally, he simplified the technique to do only what was visible and anatomically explainable. With time and boredom coming, the mind began to turn to the number of customers and money needed, to end up becoming more and more obsessed and fearful at the same time. After less than ten years, nothing remained of the original spirit or the therapeutic will.

This is why, even if we do not understand all the ins and outs, it is essential to apply to the letter the recommendations of our *Senseis*[6] who were before us on the Way. First and foremost, work daily and tirelessly on your body, your breath, your lifestyle and the quality of gestures and words. Next, question the reason that pushes us to want to touch people and even to want to help them, to check if our desire, our morals, our ethics, are correct. Finally, meditate to empty the mind and open the heart in order to perceive ourselves honestly (physically, emotionally and psychologically) in full consciousness to accept to let go of our own conditioning.

Seishin and *Shisei* are the basis of our moral conduct. If this morality is present, day after day, it strengthens the practitioner in his work, in his demeanour, and in his ability to overcome difficulties. Let us quote Ralph Waldo Emerson, American poet, essayist and philosopher of the 19th century:

> In the greatest disasters, in the greatest calamities, moral strength suddenly gives man a feeling of energy that makes that nothing is ever lost to him.[7]

Summary

1. *Shisei* indicates that inner strength is primarily physical.
2. Katas are the best way to develop a strong technique.
3. Repeating a *kata* requires mental strength and consistency.
4. *Shisei* gives the practitioner the righteousness, power and self-discipline he needs.
5. *Seishin* directs the practitioner's moral righteousness, sincerity and spiritual quality.
6. All these elements together contribute to inner strength.

16

Energy

Do you remember the Chinese saying in Chapter 7 that medicine is not as good as food? This saying has a second part that concludes 食补不如气 (*Shíbǔ bùrú qì*): "Food is not as good as *Qì*." So better than medicine and better than food, there is energy. And here we are at the heart of the matter.

There are hundreds of books trying to explain what *Ki* is (or *Qì* in Chinese or *Prana* in Sanskrit). Since the beginnings of Indian and then Chinese writing, attempts to explain this key notion as closely as possible have been numerous and many famous authors have sought to explain it. Explaining the nature of *Ki* is both possible and impossible. We can explain its creation, its modifications, its circulation, but it is difficult to understand its fundamental nature.

Eastern perception

In the Western mind, *Ki* has been translated as "energy". But the scientific definition of energy that is instilled in us from school interferes with our ability to grasp what *Ki* is in Asian culture. We think analytically and want to grasp *Ki* in a concrete, visible way, which is not the case in Asian culture. They rely on their feelings, the truth of which is as true, as consistent as, for example, a pebble or a tree. The ability to feel *Ki* is linked to the quality of our relationship with nature. But it is also hindered by the degree of scientism to which we are mentally attached. For an Asian, and especially for the ancient Chinese, Japanese, Koreans and Vietnamese, *Ki* is a fluid as concrete as water, although invisible and intangible. Invisible doesn't mean inconsistent or that you can't feel it. If you stand next to a mobile phone while it is emitting electromagnetic radiation, some can feel the waves and heat, yet you can see nothing.

The etymological reading of the kanji "Ki" allows us to better understand what it contains. Within the character, we can see several roots that are called radicals: 氣

- At the bottom the character 米 represents cooked rice; more precisely, the pictogram is that of rice tied in bales, with a string in the centre to hold them together.
- Above and on the right-hand side, these are the stylized sides of a pot.
- The slanted line above and to the left represents the raised lid of the pot.
- Finally, above it are the horizontal lines that represent the escaping steam.

To sum up the character, we can say that thanks to the cooking of rice, the steam lifts the lid. Yet the steam is intangible. Nevertheless, it is capable of lifting a metal cover and, I will even add, of moving mountains. The rice here represents food, and the pot the human body. By eating we transform food into a heat that can lift us, move us and help us progress in life. This is Ki, an invisible and impalpable steam that moves us.

Sometimes for my students, half for a laugh, half seriously, I add that the Chinese have forgotten two radicals[1] to fully understand the meaning of the character Ki: water and fire. Without fire there is no vital heat to cook food, and the rice will stay in cold water and eventually decompose into a kind of oatmeal. Without water, again cooking is not possible, or the rice will simply burn. Steam is the interaction of water and fire. These two notions remain invisible in the writing of the kanji, but they are nevertheless necessary for life. The human body is hot (37°C on average) and composed of liquids, mainly water (up to 65%). It is also the symbol of the two kidneys that are the creators of Yin/Yang. So, is this an oversight? In-depth studies of Sinology teach us to consider Chinese writing differently from what it apparently represents. The meaning is often hidden from the neophyte, and we must learn how to see what is not visible, just like Ki.

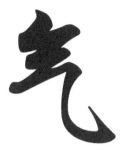

TODAY THE CHINESE CHARACTER QÌ HAS
BEEN EXTREMELY SIMPLIFIED.
THERE IS NO LONGER THE INNER PART, MEANING
THAT ENERGY RESTS ON THE VOID.

Western vision

For Westerners, the Asian notion of energy remains a mystery. Yet it is a very simple reality. But like everything that is simple, apprehending it remains complicated. However, as we have all gone to school, we have scientific references that can help us better understand this phenomenon. What forms of energy do we already know?

- **Thermal energy**: this is the oldest one we know of, historically. From the heat of the Sun, volcanoes, lightning, to that of the fire that we sought to master very early to cook, heat and protect, this form of energy is the one we know best. This energy is within us since we are warm-blooded beings. To obtain it we mix food, drink and air. Let's not forget that combustion is not possible without oxygen, so the air supply is not to be underestimated. Food and breathing are therefore the two sources of our biological heat.
- **Kinetic energy**: our body moves in space and, like everything that moves, it requires energy (we could say fuel) and also creates energy (motor energy). This form of energy is also within us because everything in the body is constantly moving: breath, blood and lymphatic circulation, intestinal transit, our muscles. Thus, we also have this kinetic energy.
- **Chemical energy**: we have all had fun in chemistry class doing experiments – more or less successfully – mixing products of

all kinds. The reactions are varied, but there is always a release of energy by contraction, expansion, cooling, heating, or even explosion. In our body, it's the same thing. Each transformation that the body makes also creates reactions that release energy. When we break down food in the stomach or molecules in the liver, or create hormones in the endocrine glands, compact stool, filter nutrients or liquids, repair the body after an accident, etc., in all these cases, we have a chemical energy constantly at work in our body.

- **Electrical energy**: pressing a button to get light is such a common gesture that we forget that a fabulous energy circulates in our homes. But our body also contains its own electrical network with the nervous system. When you step on a thorn, your brain immediately knows. You do not have to wait several seconds for a fluid to come to the brain to deliver the information. The nerve impulse is instantaneous and circulates at high speed. Every thought does the same between neurons and synapses. Our brain is the great centre of electrical impulses that organize and distribute our thoughts. So, we also have this type of energy. By the way, the human body has an electric current of 0.3 mA (milliampere); this is very useful information to understand how future integrated computer applications that the large groups of the GAFAM[2] are developing will work. IBM created a patch, stuck on the skin, that contains a personal business card, more than ten years ago now. With a simple handshake, information was exchanged, and we could know – via a computer – whom we had shaken hands with at a cocktail party. Today Google is trying to develop a contact lens that projects our emails directly onto the retina. To operate, the lens use our bioenergy.

- **Potential energy**: this form of energy is often difficult for students to understand. When you park a car on a slope, the handbrake locks the wheels. Potentially, the car can run down the slope, but in this case, it doesn't. It accumulates potential energy that can set it in motion at any time. We do the same when we sleep. We accumulate enough potential energy to get up in great shape the next morning. The key word of potential energy is "accumulation". Hence the paramount importance of having a good sleep. We can also consciously raise the potential of our energy in the middle of the day by meditating. Meditation is like flipping the handbrake. While we are on a daytime rhythm, we stop moving physically and mentally. The effect after an hour is a great inner rest. We have regained potential energy to remain peaceful, just by feeling our breathing, to better resume the course of our lives. This is why great meditators sleep so little.

- **Atomic energy:** we all know, alas, by the existence of the atomic bomb, to what extent the smallest atom conceals an energy of extraordinary power. Before being molecular beings, we are first composed of atoms, just like all the matter that surrounds us. The billions and billions of atoms that compose us rotate on themselves, fidget, shake and move continuously. We are full of this atomic energy that gives off heat and frenetic vibrations.

- **Vibrational energy**: all vibrations form waves which, as we know today, create an important and very useful energy. With this energy of the waves, we listen to the radio, watch television, converse on our mobile phones, and heat our dishes in the microwave. The photons of the Sun that warm us are both atoms and waves. Colours are waves. When we put on catchy music, we feel full of energy and work more easily, and still, this is waves. When we are depressed, we feel that we radiate less, and that the energy is no longer there. This vibratory energy is released of course by our atoms, but also by our internal movements (breathing, digestion, etc.), chemical reactions, nerve impulses, emotions and thoughts. Everything in our body is a creator of vibrations, therefore waves. However, as with radio and TV, the waves always carry a signal, a message, information.

To conclude, Westerners have divided energy into different categories thanks to analytical science. In Asian culture, all this is one and the same. The *Ki* of the ancient Asians is nothing but the sum of all the energies we know of, but instead of dissecting it, they conceive it as a whole, a package if you will. Westerners have separated the different manifestations of energy because they are observable and analysable. The Asians have preserved its unity so as not to separate themselves from nature. And therefore, they are correct in saying that Ki is everywhere, that it circulates from the cosmos into our cells, constantly creates movement and yet remains essentially invisible.

Origins of energy

In the Chinese Classics, universal energy comes from Heaven. To say precisely what this energy is, what its form is, its nature, is akin to discussing the sex of angels. Is it the light of the Sun, of all the stars, the rotational motion of our galaxy, the dark matter of the universe, gravity and gravitational waves, space-time, whatever? For the human species, it is above all the energy that comes from above and touches us. The ancient Chinese referred to it as Heaven and spoke of its Yang nature. The Earth receives this energy from Heaven, absorbs it, matures it, transforms it to send it back to Heaven in a different form. Our planet is a living organism, from the single-celled amoeba to the great currents of the oceans, from the cycle of oxygen through that of water, from the internal movement of its nucleus to that of the layers of the atmosphere, from the succession of seasons to the succession of lives, everything is life and movement.

Between Heaven and Earth are three kingdoms: mineral, vegetable and animal, of which the human being is only one of the species, even if it sometimes perceives itself as a species apart because of its intellect. The minerals are the basis of our earthly life and absorb heat and radiation of all kinds. They are also able to return this energy, as do radioactive minerals for example. The vegetable kingdom feeds on the minerals and gathers their essence. It also uses light and waves, plus air and water. This life is therefore more complex and consumes more energy. The herbivorous animals feed on plants and absorb their essence as well as the essence of the minerals they incorporated, not to mention light, waves, air and water. The carnivorous animals feed on the herbivores and thus absorb the three kingdoms, without forgetting everything else, plus instincts and emotions. As for the omnivorous man, he absorbs absolutely everything. He is the result of all kingdoms, by direct or indirect absorption, and therefore integrates all the previous energies. He transforms this nourishment to adapt it to his needs. For this, he also uses air, water, light, waves, instincts, emotions, and adds thought. All this forms the energy of his body and mind, energy that he creates and spends constantly. As the Chinese say, 人活一口气 (*Rén huó yī kǒu qì*): Men live mainly on energy.

The Classics of Chinese medicine name up to 36 different forms of energy in the body, but to simplify we can say that there is the energy of air 空气 (*Kōng qì*), food 骨气 (*Gǔ qì*) and the inheritance from ancestors via the original energy 元气 (*Yuán qì*). As they blend together, they will create the true *Ki* 正气 (*Zhèng qì*). This will be divided into two major functions: the defensive energy 卫气 (*Wèi qì*) which protects the body against pathologies and climatic aggressions, and the nourishing energy 营气 (*Yíng qì*) which sustains the whole organism via the Blood 血 (*Xuè*). Blood according to the Chinese vision is the binder, the common asset of the whole organism, both red liquid and materialized energy.

Understanding all this allows several things. First, from a global point of view, it is to realize that everything that composes us is only energy, from space to our atoms. Second, from the point of view of quality of life, human energy is the result of a diet through which Man captures the essence of all living things. This is why the wise man pays attention to what he eats and knows the relationship he has with his environment since its fruits enter him and constitute him. Finally, from a therapeutic point of view, knowing the overall pattern of the different types of *Qì* makes it possible to act more precisely on internal imbalances. For the Shiatsu practitioner, this is also a good way to guide the advice he can give. If the *Yíng qì* is affected, these tips will focus on diet and sleep. If *Wèi qì* is affected, it will encourage strengthening the body through energetic exercise, heat and eating certain foods. These are, of course, just a few examples.

Energy circulation

As we have seen, the universal *Ki* flows from Heaven to Earth, and returns in the opposite direction after being transformed. This direction of circulation indicates that there is an order of things, a precedence of Heaven. The information comes from the top to go down and inform the bottom. It carries its message, whatever it is. This is the principle of Yang (阳), the macrocosm, designated in Chinese by three superimposed horizontal solid lines (☰), same as the number three. These three solid lines also symbolize Heaven, Man and Earth, indicating that from the start Yang contains the organization of the whole and even of the microcosm. The more the Yang descends, the more matter is created. For its part, Earth receives the Yang within it. This is the Yin principle (阴), represented by three superimposed lines (☷), but these lines are broken, to let the light of Heaven pass through, to welcome in order to be fertilized. This ontological fissure allows the creation of life. Life then unfolds on its surface and tends to rise towards Yang.

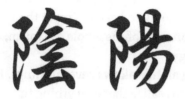

IN/YŌ IN JAPANESE OR YIN/YANG IN CHINESE, THE TWO PRINCIPLES AT THE FOUNDATIONS OF ALL LIFE.

Man – like all forms of life that walk on Earth – continually receives the influences of celestial Yang and terrestrial Yin. These two forces pass through him to animate him. Given the complexity of his body, his emotions and his psyche, Qì is divided into many forms – or vibrations – to provide him with the throughput he needs to exist. Answering its dual Yin/Yang nature, human Qì is divided into two types. The first energetic form is Jīng (精 – translated as "Essence" but meaning "refined"). This forms the structure of the body, its development and its eight directions (up–down, right–left, front–back, inside–surface). The Jīng moves slowly via the eight Extraordinary Meridians 奇经八脉 (Qí jīng bā mài), on a cycle of seven years for women and eight years for men. It manages the major stages of life. The second energetic form is true Qì (itself divided into Wèi qì of Yang nature and Yíng qì of Yin nature), which allows human activity, movement, creation, complexity of thought, etc. This true Qì circulates rapidly in the 12 main meridians (also called "ordinary" in comparison to the "extraordinary" meridians) over a 24-hour cycle. The link between Essence and *Qì* goes through the Kidney, which serves as both a storage and an engine capable of transforming *Qì* into *Jīng* and vice versa. All this is widely studied in Shiatsu schools and even more so in Chinese medicine schools, so I will not elaborate further.[3]

For a *shiatsushi*, the most important thing is to know and understand these two energy forms. If we add to this transportation channels and points 経穴 (*keiketsu* in Japanese, acupuncture points), he will know what to do to help a client. For example, if you are facing a growth problem in a child, there is no point in stimulating the meridians (except for the Kidney), because the heart of the problem concerns the Extraordinary Meridians. On the other hand, for constipation, the Extraordinary Meridians will be of less help than the Large Intestine and Lung meridians.

Vibration of energy

One of the main concerns for Shiatsu students is the following question: "How to feel the energy in the meridians and how to be sure that it is *Qì*?" Let's start with a statement that can be tricky to grasp: as long as we ask ourselves this question it is difficult to feel the energy, unless we have a special gift as is the case for some people. It certainly takes time to develop the hands' sensitivity, but it is essential to let go of the analytical mind to get in touch with *Qì*. Indeed, as long as the mind is questioning, we hear nothing from what the hands and even the rest of the body feel. This is usually where scientific minds pick up and laugh, because they assume that there is a trick. But no one said that we could not have an analytical mind about energy. You just can't do both at once. We must first feel the subtle and then, only then, it will be possible to move on to the analysis of what was felt. The day an ungifted student – as I was – contacts the flow of energy, he knows it instantly and instinctively without being able to explain how he knows it. It is obvious, a revelation that usually brings a lot of smiles, emotions, laughter and sometimes even tears of joy. It can be frustrating to lose this sensation, but facing the loss of control the mind comes back to spread doubt on all levels. Do not worry. It will come back by dint of listening, patience, trust and inner silence. Don't believe! Don't believe anything! *Ki* is not a religion and does not require prayer or special faith. Live according to the principles of a healthy and inner life, then the sensations will return to never leave you.

As noted before, energy vibrates. Every atom, every molecule, every cell, every mitochondrion, every bacteria, every pulse of blood, every emotion, every thought, every movement creates a vibration. With experience, the practitioner realizes that each meridian vibrates differently. The Liver's biological rhythm is very slow; its meridian does not vibrate at the same speed as the Heart, for example. Furthermore, the Yin or Yang nature of the meridians makes them vibrate at very different tempos as well. Over time, he will also discover the vibrations induced by disturbances in the circulation of energy 邪气 (Xiéqi) or "perverse energy". A blockage (Fullness) does not vibrate in the same way as an absence of energy (Emptiness). To be sure that the feeling cannot be confused with something else, the best approach is to proceed in the following way: feel different areas of the body where you can take the pulse (wrist, under the left breast, jugular artery, ankle, etc.). Learning to take the radial pulse and feel its many variations also allows you to refine your feelings. After five or ten minutes of silence, the student is encouraged to describe what he perceived. But what he will describe can have many explanations, so I recommend drawing the variation of the energy in the air with a finger (or on a board with a marker). Starting from the basic principle that a balanced energy rises and falls with regularity, it can be represented in the form of a sinusoid. From there, the exercise becomes easy. If it stings like needles in the fingers, the energy is too excited. We can then, like a seismograph, bring the sinusoidal curves closer together until it looks like peaks. If it sizzles under the fingers, it may indicate low and intermittent energy, much like the filament of a bulb at the end of its life. We would draw a flattened curve but shaken by crackling. No energy: a flat line drawn at the bottom of the chart. An electric shock in the fingers: the energy is blocked and looking for a way out. The curve is flat and agitated but it would be drawn at the top of the chart. By developing this sort of system, it becomes easy to represent the feeling of energy and to communicate, compare, exchange between the student and the teacher. Thus, the student will be accompanied, guided; he will be able to use the same yardstick as his teacher and will gain confidence in the certainty that he is now touching the Grail, the feeling of Qì.

Living with Ki

Philosophically speaking, *Ki* is the energy that flows between Heaven and Earth. This fluid is found in everything, transforms and transports everything. Without it there is no life, change or movement. Man in his role as a conductive wire must circulate this energy in the best possible conditions. This is why he must ensure the good condition of his meridians, his internal channels for energy circulation. That is his task. His mission. The number 3 or the symbol of Yang that we saw previously is drawn with three superimposed lines that symbolize Heaven, Man and Earth. As soon as Man rises between Heaven and Earth, his line becomes vertical and connects the other two horizontal lines. The character "three" changes meaning and becomes the character 工 (*gōng*), which means "to work". Thus, the only real work of Man is to straighten up to connect Heaven and Earth.

To be fully connected to *Ki*, a *shiatsushi* accepts his work of being human, aware of his task and responsibility. For this he knows, understands and feels his fundamental energy channels (the Extraordinary Meridians), secondary channels (the main meridians) and his general communication network (the *Luò* meridians). He listens to himself from within, harmonizes the flows, regulates his breath, lifts his physical, mental and emotional blockages. That is his primary role. His secondary role is to help people live without blockage to help Yin/Yang meet, blend harmoniously and transmute.

Living in and with *Ki* is not easy. It is a daily discipline, listening every moment, a choice of life. It is a demanding Way that requires regularity and study, intellect and feeling without thought, Emptiness and Fullness, understanding the principles of life according to its different rhythms (hour, day, month, season, year, cycle of *Jīng* in seven or eight years depending on sex, Five Elements, Yin and Yang). The easiest way to work in this field is to stop one or more times during the day and look inwards by asking yourself a few questions: How am I doing overall? What about my intestines? And my breathing? What about my digestion? What about my emotions? Is my diet correct and does it meet my needs? Do my desires take precedence over my needs? We will start from the whole to go onto the details. We can possibly palpate to feel more, but normally simple introspection allows us to quickly know where we are. Under no circumstances should you look for the answers in your brain, otherwise it will quickly conclude that everything is fine and that you should not bother. No. You must listen, touch, feel, move with the breath.

Far from the idea of living like a monk and taking a vow of abstinence, it is important to continue to live fully because it is exciting to live. You can even have fun with Ki, play and do tricks that always amaze those around you. I love doing this and demonstrating how easy it is to laugh with energy. When I do public demonstrations or sometimes during workshops, I show a few tricks, and everyone cheers up and laughs like children. It's normal! Discovery is a primary joy for children. To play with energy, try this exercise. Ask a person to bend their forearm at a right angle, fist closed with the index finger stretched forward. To contract the arm in this way, it is the meridian of the Large Intestine that works. Press both your hands on their fist to lower the arm. Normally the person resists quite well thanks to his biceps. Now put your thumb or index finger on GI 20, wait two or three seconds to feel the energy of this point, then with the other hand lower the fist again. Impossible for the person to resist. There are dozens of small games to do like this to have fun in class and become aware of the reality of Ki.

The difference between before and after the exercise is that, after, everything happens mindfully. To feel Ki, we must above all accept to surrender, forget our Cartesian and materialistic mental constructions and let ourselves be guided by instinct and intuition, go beyond our beliefs in scientific rationalism to address the non-verbal communication of nature. It is a long and exciting journey in and towards oneself with nothing less than the understanding of the universe (macrocosm and microcosm) and the mechanisms of life (inner and outer) and the mind (mind and universal consciousness) at stake. Whenever we feel a blockage, a tightness, a muscular knot, a psychological tension, we will stop there to study them, identify them, find their causes and their relationships with all dimensions of the human being (body–mind–emotions–soul). As appropriate, we will try to untie, dissolve, circulate, reheat, cool to finally forget and return to a state of equilibrium. Once again, the less the mind gets involved, the more we remain present to the sensitive reality of the body. But we will help ourselves by guiding the breath to the area under tension, with a gentle and loving intention. Then *Ki* flows in and out of oneself and will allow the *shiatsushi* to fulfil his mission.

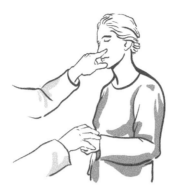

DO THIS MUSCLE RESISTANCE TEST WITH AND WITHOUT
CONNECTION TO THE TRIGGERED MERIDIAN.
THE DIFFERENCE IS STAGGERING!

Summary

1. *Ki* is the energy that underlies the whole universe, life and movement of life.
2. Whatever the vision (Eastern or Western), we all recognize the existence of energy on all planes of existence.
3. *Ki* is divided into two forms: Yin and Yang, which are inseparable.
4. Yang comes from Heaven and goes to Earth, then goes back the other way in the form of Yin.
5. The human body circulates *Jīng* in eight Extraordinary Meridians, and true *Qì* in 12 meridians.
6. The vibration of energy in the meridians can be felt and indicates the quality or imbalance in the energy circulation.

Emptiness and Excess

Zero, in Old Chinese
Tiny space between raindrops
Mystery of the Void. [1]

As we have seen, the circulation of *Ki* or *Qì* energy through the human body emanates from a natural phenomenon between the two great primordial polarities: Heaven and Earth. But between these two powers, the human being sometimes fails to find the correct flow of energy. He then lives between small misfortunes and glorious waves or, we might say, between grandeur and decadence. The Japanese who closely study the meridians speak of *kyo* and *jitsu*, energy Emptiness and its opposite, Fullness.

The reasons for blockages

There are many disturbances of the harmonious flow of energy, and the human being seems to be the all-round champion for creating new ones every day. As the common thread of Yin/Yang, his task is not easy. Everything we experience can potentially change the flow of the celestial breath. If we make a census of the reasons that lead us to disturbed energy, we realize that the list is almost endless. However, it can be summarized as follows, in no order of importance or preference:

- Traumatic accidents
- Weather disturbances

- Poor diet
- An excess of activities without sufficient rest
- Lack of physical exercise
- Poor emotional management
- Excessive mental activity
- Negative thoughts
- Medications and their side effects
- Infections and parasites of the body
- The absence or excess of social relations
- Excessive sexual relations
- Electronic disturbances (waves)
- Pollution (air, agricultural, industrial, etc.).

Ki is so sensitive that it takes very little to upset it. As I have told you, I often show, during public demonstrations, small games that are very visual and that obviously show energy, so that they can see the effects on the human body. One of these games is to disrupt the flow of *Ki* in the arms with simple paper handkerchiefs, which halves muscle strength. If pieces of paper can alter the flow of *Ki*, imagine what a mobile phone can do. This reminds me of an oncologist who told me that X-rays now show rectangular tumours, exactly the shape of the owner's mobile phone when it is constantly carried in a pocket against the body. Makes you think.

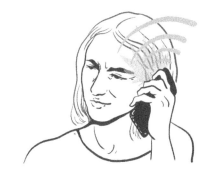

MOBILE PHONE MICROWAVES DISRUPT OUR
ENERGY IN AN IMPRESSIVE WAY.
JUST DO RESISTANCE TESTS WITH AND WITHOUT
A LIVE PHONE ON IN ONE HAND.

Rereading the previous list, we see that the words "absence" and "excess" come up. And for good reason! If everything remains balanced, in homeostasis, there is no reason for the circulation of *Ki* in the meridians to change. If, on the other hand, excess sets in (for example, too much chocolate every day), the body must immediately adapt to this overload. For this, the digestive organs will call on more *Ki* in the Spleen-Pancreas. But this increase in *Ki* in one place means that *Ki* will be taken from another organ, which will weaken it. Remember that all relationships between organs are dynamic thanks to the circulation of *Ki*. But if one blocks *Ki* in one organ to cope with an excess, then another organ will suffer. In other words, the meridians will have to compensate for each other, which will at one time or another influence the tissues and organs of the body. This is why any excess is harmful. The reverse is also true. If in your diet you never receive any iron intake, you will go straight towards anaemia. Absence is therefore just as harmful as excess.

These notions of Emptiness and excess are the basis of Eastern medicine, and they are found everywhere in the founding book of Chinese medicine, *The Yellow Emperor's Classic of Medicine* (*Huángdì Nèijīng*). Here are just two examples among dozens:

- Chapter 10:
  "Headache with dementia: there is Void below and Fullness above. The evil is in the Shaoyin and the foot Taiyang. In case of aggravation, it penetrates the kidneys."
  是以頭痛巔疾. 下虛上實. 過在足少陰巨陽. 甚則入腎.
- Chapter 28:
  "The Emperor: The pulses of madness, what about them in terms of Emptiness and Fullness?"
  帝曰. 癲疾何如. 岐伯曰. 脈搏大滑. 久自已. 脈小堅急. 死不治.
  "Qi Bo: If they are empty, it can heal; If they are full, it is death."
  帝曰. 癲疾之脈. 虛實何如. 岐伯曰. 虛則可治. 實則死.

The three disorders

Shiatsu students all over the world are familiar with the following disturbances, at least the first two, because they were greatly popularized by Shizuto Masunaga.[2] The following terms are therefore in Japanese.

Kyo 虚

This is the notion of Emptiness that is found in Oriental medicine. When a meridian is lacking energy, partially or completely, it is said to be *kyo*. We can easily recognize this state by feeling an absence of tonicity of the surface tissues first, then in the muscles. It forms like a small depression under the finger. There is often cold, although not always, and the *jusha* says that it does him good when pressed. The reason is simple: deep pressure brings the warmth and energy it lacks. Therefore, we can conclude that *kyo* is an absence of *Ki*.

Jitsu 実

This is the opposite notion, excess. In Oriental medicine, they speak of Fullness. It is also quite easy to find because the tissues are hard, there is tension and a resistance to pressure, pressure that cannot immediately pass through. Heat is often found, although not all the time, because it takes a lot of energy in one place on the body to create a blockage. The *jusha* complains that pressure is painful when the *shiatsushi*'s fingers are on it.

Teitai 停滞

Those who have not studied Oriental medicine are here faced with a third notion that is not necessarily seen in Shiatsu: Stagnation. This is classically considered as another form of Fullness. In fact, Stagnation is not the absence or excess of energy. There is energy, but it does not flow. This situation is quite common and often precedes Emptiness or Fullness depending on the case. For example, a simple thought or an emotion can very quickly stagnate the *Ki* in an organ, frequently the Liver who is quite customary of the fact. If *Ki* is not quickly put back into circulation, the situation is likely to degenerate into *kyo* or *jitsu*, depending on the circumstances. Stagnation can be identified by the fact that it forms a hard plate in the tissues, like an obstruction, more or less painful depending on the place and the person. Stasis is neither full nor empty but gives the impression of a blockage. Moreover, we feel little or no activity in the stasis area, and this is normal since nothing circulates.

These three energy disturbances must be known by heart, because they require an appropriate response. During a first treatment with a woman in her fifties, I could not find the pulse of the Liver. It can happen, I wasn't properly awake, and I started my treatment without thinking about it any more. She had come with a very clear request for back pain. After 45 minutes, I finally touched the liver while working on the *hara*. Surprise, the liver was completely flat, flaccid, without resistance. I could literally push the entire length of my fingers under the right ribs. "How are you feeling psychologically right now?" I asked. "I'm not feeling good, I feel depressed, I have no energy, no desire and everything weighs on me. In short, I have had enough of this life." I had missed a complete void in the pulse of the Liver, the organ was in Blood Deficiency, the Hun (Spirit of the Liver) no longer brought imagination. The back was the symptom, the cause was the Liver. I treated this person for eight months before her imagination and lust for life timidly returned. As soon as she regained her strength, she left her job, her husband and the country, to live under the sun of Portugal. Today if I do not feel a pulse, my senses are immediately alert. That was a lesson for me.

Tonification and dispersal

The previous concepts are very real, and it is important to know how to regulate them in order to avoid the appearance of further symptoms. Excesses are overflows of energy that form agitation and blockages in the body. If you do not know how to treat them, it is quite possible to stimulate them more and therefore increase the problems. This is why all Shiatsu students, after the first year, must know the techniques for dispersing and tonifying.

Ho 補

This is the tonifying principle. It is applied to a *kyo* (empty) place to regenerate it. The translation of the kanji, radical and character, means "clothing" and "to glue a piece". Literally, it is "repairing a garment with a piece of the same fabric". The cloth in question is of course *Ki*. Several techniques exist to tonify a Void, it depends on the school. The most common techniques are:

- leave the hand or finger for a long time, deep in the depression with a sustained attention that seeks to fill the Void, until one feels the area plump gently under the finger
- press and rotate clockwise with a finger in the empty area
- in addition, moxibustion can be used if it is an empty point, or a Chinese lamp (*Wai qì*) if it is a larger area.

Shā 寫

This is the principle of dispersion. Applied to *jitsu* (Full) or *teitai* (Stasis) points. The kanji is interesting. It represents a horse (we can see the four legs at the bottom) carrying a package closed by a lid, hence its meaning of "transfer, move to, dump". The most common Shiatsu[3] techniques for dispersing are:

- press repeatedly on the point, without much force
- press and turn counterclockwise on the excess area with a finger
- open the extremities (fingers and toes) to chase away energy according to the flow.

Masunaga speaks of *Ho sha* as two techniques that are not isolated. As said before, where there is an excess, a vacuum is created elsewhere. He is perfectly right in this, moreover in the *Lingshu*, in Chapter 75, we can read these words from the mouth of the Minister Qi Bo: "Emptiness is an insufficiency, and Fullness is an overabundance. Light and heavy do not match."

Masunaga was an intellectual trained in psychology and Shiatsu. He knew classical medicine very well, which is why he stated that the *Ho sha* technique consists in transferring the overflow to the empty area, to regulate and then harmonize the *tsubos*, areas or channels, so that they regain their balance and dynamic movement.

However, the *Ho sha* technique presupposes that all the energy a person needs is already in him since we start from the principle of transferring an excess to a void. Clinical practice shows that this is not always true. A person can be in a state of generalized Emptiness, as with burn-out or a serious illness, without the slightest resource in any corner of the body to rebalance himself. Oriental medicine then explains that it is also necessary to know how to regenerate a person. This is where pharmacopoeia, diet and moxibustion come in. But for us Shiatsu practitioners, it is the principle of *Ki musubi* (see Chapter 22) that will link the energy of the practitioner to that of the patient and to carry out an energy transfer. The practitioner must obviously know all the dietary and lifestyle recommendations, as well as exercises to help the person rebuild.

Summary

1. *Kyo* and *jitsu* are the two key concepts of energy imbalance. One represents the state of Emptiness and the other that of Fullness (excess).
2. *Ki* is so sensitive that the slightest disturbance can alter or weaken it.
3. There are three types of *Ki* disruption, Emptiness, Fullness and Stagnation. You must know what you can do to resolve these situations.
4. The *Ho sha* technique involves transferring the excess to an empty area or *tsubo*.

18

Overall Vision

Prevailing alone
Against the autumn sky
The Mount Fuji

TAIGU RYOKAN (1758–1831)

A t the beginning of a session, while the recipient enters the Shiatsu practice, walks, sits, talks or lies down, the practitioner observes, listens, notes, smells and feels. He pays attention to visible details and invisible signs. He listens to what is said and hears what is not uttered. He sees the appearance of the outer body and seeks to understand what is at stake inside. It is said that he sees far, beyond appearances. The Japanese expression *enzan'no metsuke* (遠山の目付) captures this idea of seeing globally, a landscape for example, without forgetting anything, but without focusing on all the details. The expression literally means "to see the whole as one sees the mountain in the distance", which is shortened to "to look at a distant mountain". It is a question of adopting a vision that is present and absent at the same time, which allows us both to see the individual movements and to paint a general picture without attaching oneself to the myriad of details that come up.

Learning to observe without seeing

To understand this concept, here is a little exercise: observe an entire field, a city, a mountain, a crowd or a face, but without focusing on the details. A bit like being myopic and without your glasses. The gaze does not concern itself with details but favours a general perception. One might think that the practitioner is daydreaming or absent, but on the contrary, he is very present, paying attention to the movements and the different nuances of the body. This state makes it possible to capture the general picture of the person, while revealing some useful details that would not be visible if he focused directly on a specific detail.

The founder of Aikidō, O Sensei Morihei Ueshiba, recommended to his disciples the following principles:

> Do not look at the eyes of *aite* 相手 ["opponent or partner"], the heart is drawn in by the eyes of *aite*; Do not look at the sword of *aite*, the spirit is drawn in by the sword of *aite*; Do not look at *aite*, you'd let the *Ki* of *aite* in. The Bu 武 [here in the sense of "battle"] of truth is an exercise in attracting the adversary in his entirety.[1]

Therefore, observing without seeing, being present without focusing on anything, is the only solution in a combat situation. It is interesting to see that in Aikidō the notion of an invasive *Ki* is mistaken. This recommendation is also valid for the *shiatsushi* because the *Ki* of the *jusha* can quickly run into him and transmit his problems and symptoms.

For his part, Ohashi Sensei shows that it is sometimes difficult to see what is wrong with a person because our eyes capture too many details. To see better, you must conceal the person. For this, he covers the person under a light, fluid sheet. By obliterating the details in this way, the essential stands out: we can clearly see the bumps and hollows, the folds of the sheet indicate the lines of tension and the height differences of the barriers (shoulders, hips, etc.), as well as everything that malfunctions in the posture of the body. This technique is a way of "looking into the distance" to know the general picture of a postural problem.

This general attention to the recipient's body also makes it possible to capture details as part of a whole. In practice, the recipient can tell you that his head hurts. While the practitioner pays attention to the person, he hears the slightly whiny timbre of the voice that indicates that his situation is painful, he sees the swollen temporal vein that pulsates and shows a disorder in blood circulation, the somewhat red complexion of the face that specifies a rise of Yang or the presence of Heat, the movement of the hand that instinctively designates the area the pain is coming from, the posture of the back that can show the state of the Kidney, the brightness of the eye where the *Shén* 神 (Spirit) shines; he smells the sweat, sees the tiny trembling of the limbs, and so on.

If the practitioner focuses on a specific detail or looks for a particular one, he will not see the others or the general picture. This is also the drama of current Western medicine that has difficulty remaining holistic. Looking at nothing in particular, a thousand and one details arise in the practitioner's empty mind. He then effortlessly notes the information that comes to him, and a general drawing appears, a backstory unfolds. Thus, he can choose a treatment strategy that will be in line with everything he has perceived.

Sight and movement

Our gaze also directs our movements. It is the eye that orientates and directs the body or the hand, gives the direction to follow. We are so used to watching where we are going – except for the distracted ones – that it would not occur to us to have a broader vision to free our movements. Most people walking in the street look straight ahead or at their feet (to avoid dog droppings or to avoid meeting the eyes of their peers). But if an obstacle arises, they are stuck. They then look for another way by looking right and left. Martial arts practitioners can be spotted in the street by the way they look up and as widely as possible to the sides, up and down, in front of them and in depth. If a danger presents itself on their sidewalk, such as a shady individual for example, they feel and listen to their instincts and change direction or sidewalk long before they have to face a potentially perilous situation. This way of opening one's eyes to everything that happens is a great advantage for one's safety and during combat.

Shiatsu does not fight anything. It balances and soothes. Nevertheless, the principles of this manual technique are the same as in martial arts. When we watch students practising, we see that they are looking with all their strength at the area or point they are pressing, as if they were trying to see what is happening underneath. As we cannot see under the surface of a body with our eyes, it is useless. At the start, the first few months, this can be reassuring for the position of the fingers and the accuracy of their location, but it is better to get rid of it quickly. It could become a bad habit, especially because you lower your head and constantly stretch the neck muscles. One of my former students always complained about not feeling anything, not finding anything, that he wasn't any good, that Shiatsu was not for him. I noticed that he was always completely strained because of his gaze fixed on the precise place where he put his fingers. When I blindfolded him with a *tenugui* and asked him to redo the points, he discovered another dimension and said: "It's as if I'm seeing for the first time." After that, I made him contemplate landscapes in the countryside, to learn to "see without seeing". Once he became a practitioner, he admitted to me that he did entire sessions with his eyes closed just for pleasure.

But, above all, closing your eyes allows you to see the inner landscapes of a person by improving sensations. However, if we observe a Shiatsu master during his practice, his gaze is in the distance, half-closed, as if he were elsewhere. The reason is as follows: placing the gaze at a specific place fixes the body and hands at that place and often creates a phenomenon of attraction, a concentration that causes a delay or hampers free movement around the body of the recipient. A beginner may look at his fingers, but an advanced *shiatsushi* must get over this stage because, as the Chinese saying goes: "When the master points to the moon, the idiot looks at the finger." The master who does not look at anything in particular can go where he wants. He is freer in his movements, his hands know by heart the human body, channels and *tsubos*, so he can focus on his feelings. In addition, he navigates between inner sensations and external observation, never a prisoner of appearances or feelings only.

Observing to learn better

To get used to seeing beyond, the first thing is, I repeat myself, to not look at your fingers, at least not all the time. Among the different stages of the education of young *shiatsushi*, this one is relatively simple to request and implement. With a little practice, the gaze detaches from the fingers and the feeling increases. In addition, this open gaze is useful to learn the essence of what the teacher is showing. The Japanese term *mitori geiko* means "to capture the technique" or "to learn with the gaze". As long as the beginner looks at the hands of the teacher, he does not see that the essence of the technique is not there. The essentials usually go unnoticed: spatial movement, feet placement, distance managing, the permanent attention necessary for the proper realization of a technique. If the student's attention is on the teacher's fingers, he will know how to place his fingers soon enough but not much will happen. He will try and try again without being able to succeed in his movement. On the other hand, if the student looks globally at the teacher's body, he will capture everything that builds the technique. His finger placement will probably be less precise, but he will manage to trigger a correct pressure that will immediately have an effect. Accuracy then becomes secondary. If his teacher is vigilant, he will come to correct him. Otherwise, the student will always be able to study the precise location of the *tsubos* once he gets home or is in a revision group.

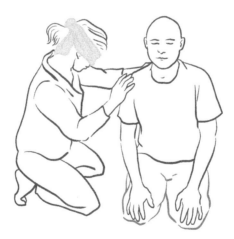

VOLUNTARILY DEPRIVING ONESELF OF SIGHT ALLOWS ONE
TO DEVELOP THE SENSES OF TOUCH AND FEELING.

As for more or less experienced practitioners, working without look-ing is an excellent exercise and I encourage all *shiatsushi* to perform long parts of their sessions with their eyes closed or blindfolded during a class. Then, senses develop, feeling increases and we can reopen our eyes without seeing a particular detail, but all the details at the same time. The *shiatsushi* will then see the eyebrows of the *jusha* contract - a sign of pain that he does not want to express - or the long exhalation that indicates letting go or a foot moving back to its place. As for his hands, they will tell him everything he cannot see with his eyes. As the famous Miyamoto Musashi wrote, "perception is strong and eyesight is weak".[2]

In the traditional education of the Far East, the notion of pedagogy does not exist. On the other hand, in learning a trade or art, training often begins with several months of observation. In Shiatsu, in old schools the students are still asked to spend days or months observing the Sensei. The advice of the master only concerns the way to look or rather to observe the whole movement, the posture of the body, the movement and the origin of the intention (of course invisible). To see the intention of a movement, one must dispense with sight, which is useless here. It is the Little Prince of Saint-Exupéry who said - with reason - that "it is only with one's heart that one can see clearly".[3]

In other words, we must get rid of the sight that sees in favour of the sight that perceives. Thus, the practitioner short-circuits the mind, the rational brain, in favour of shorter and more instantaneous circuits that are our reptilian brains and nervous circuits. The heart (understood to mean the emotions but also the spirit) also plays a big role, as we will see later on, in Chapter 26. Just as in meditation with a vague gaze,[4] the practitioner no longer thinks. Then the body of the recipient speaks directly to the body of the practitioner, who reacts accordingly, without the need to intellectualize. The intellectual phase is possibly useful only at the beginning, during diagnosis. Afterwards, he lets his hands act long before thinking about what he should do, which is a form of meditation in motion. Then he leaves, without a trace.

> Our life in this world?
> A boat that sculled away
> At the break of dawn
> Leaving no wake[5]

Summary

1. Looking globally without focusing on a detail allows you to see the general picture, the whole person.
2. Global observation makes it possible to be undisturbed and to remain serene.
3. If the gaze is open and faraway, the body moves freely.
4. Global observation makes it possible to see the essence of what the teacher is presenting.
5. Global observation offers the means to develop one's senses and to feel clearly.

19

Vigilance

Through overall observation and relaxation, the body becomes receptive and the mind empty. These two aspects go hand in hand, but they are only a stepping stone to overall vigilance. In Japanese, the term *zanshin* 残心 perfectly coveys this idea of continuous attention.

Abandoning thought

As always, the study of Japanese kanji allows us to grasp the spirit behind the words. If the term *zanshin* is commonly used to refer to "continuous attention" or "continuing attention", the literal translation is rich in teaching since *zanshin* first means "to abandon the mind". In other words, this term informs us that to be attentive the practitioner must abandon his mind (in the sense of mental activity, that of the brain). For a Western mind, this is often a contradiction that logic cannot resolve. Indeed, how can we become attentive if we abandon the brain, how can we be attentive if we do not concentrate with all our strength? Once again, this contradiction stems from our upbringing. At school and at home we were told to be careful, to follow what is happening, to listen without moving, to observe by opening our eyes wide, not to miss a crumb of events... Does this bring back memories? And when we did not behave, the teacher complained to the parents that the child is not there, is not present, is not trying. This way of considering attention has a historical origin: the philosopher René Descartes. With his famous maxim *cogito ergo sum* ("I think therefore I am"), this philosopher shaped the whole of

Western society by putting the mind at the forefront of human activity. Everything else was abject. In this he is the worthy heir of Catholic dogma[1] which states that the body is dirty, secondary, degrading, and the spirit is the means to attain the pure, the divine, the whole. Current school education has still not emerged from this diktat of thought as the only way to go beyond a physical dimension.[2] Children must be constantly present to what is being said and written on the blackboard. And this is only possible through an over-solicitation of the mind. In addition, they are forced to sit for many hours on a chair, moving as little as possible, which, is by the way – at an age when the body develops and for this very reason, is overflowing with energy – a mechanical and energetic aberration as well as an ignorance of psycho-corporal development. Everywhere in nature, animal young play; they move to develop their bodies and reflexes, as well as to live and learn about the world. Conclusion: young humans who have just finished university already have back pain and can no longer relax or sleep as the mind has been "muscled" for more than 20 years.

The Oriental way that favours the traditional learning of arts and crafts can be considered as an anti-Cartesian system. Moreover, the Eastern spirit says: "When I no longer think, I am." It is not advised to analyse but to observe and absorb. There is no point in bashing what the master says, but to experience it in ones' flesh. No need to discourse theoretically but rather discover the depths of the technique by the body. Do not learn by heart, but learn by the body. One could therefore rightly reverse the Cartesian principle by declaring: "I am, therefore I act. So, I think." Everyone will agree on the fact that to be able to think, you must first be, exist, have a body and a brain, otherwise you don't get very far. But millennia of observation of the human mind have made it possible to understand that as long as the brain remains active, the body cannot access the depth of physical experience. Thoughts block feeling and introspection. For Asian masters it is quite the opposite. The principle could then be stated as follows: "I am, therefore I feel and eventually I think," but this last part is far from obligatory because it detaches us again from the state of nature. The term *zanshin* is now clearer. It is necessary to abandon there – here and now – the mind to live the experience of the body with all the required attention.

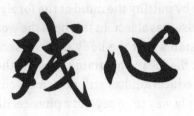

Continuous vigilance

But how does abandoning the mind allow greater vigilance? The study of brain activity by fMRI (functional MRI) in recent years has allowed better understanding of the effects of meditation on an individual. It has been observed that when a specialist concentrates on a subject he has a lot of knowledge on, he uses about 70 to 75 per cent of his neural capacity. On the other hand, when a seasoned meditator empties his mind, thinks about nothing, those same abilities reach between 85 to 90 per cent of his neural capacity. For scientists this was quite a surprise. They had just discovered that by ceasing the activity of the mind, the brain becomes much more active. Instead of concentrating (the exact meaning is "to reduce one's field of thought") the brain flourishes by exploring more and more connections through its synapses and neurons. In other words, the meditator regains possession of more of his abilities. Thanks to this first step, scientists soon discovered the plasticity of the brain. Its connections are constantly evolving and thus we can learn throughout our lives by creating new connections. This is why abandoning the mind makes it possible to apprehend much more than concentration achieves.

The rest becomes simple to understand. The Japanese have an expression that works by analogy: to calm down is to "empty the bowl". Here the bowl represents the brain. This is a funny little Japanese tale: A young man wishes to become a disciple of a famous tea master. He introduces himself according to the rules and then he begins to tell his journey. He talks about all his experiences, all his learnings, the fact that he has already attended many masters and that he is not a beginner in the art of tea and that he is sure that he will be able to bring many things to his future master. The latter, without saying a word, listens for more than an hour. He puts a cup in front of the candidate and serves him tea but does not stop once the cup is full. Very quickly the tea overflows and spreads. He then says: "How could a cup receive more tea if it was already full?" The candidate then discovers that he is constantly encumbered with what he has learned.

If the bowl is full, it cannot receive new information, because the mind is already occupied. On the other hand, if the bowl is empty, it can accommodate any new information that arises. The emptier the bowl, the more information it can receive, including the most subtle, the finest, the information not usually perceived when the mind is bubbling. The state of alertness is reached. Vigilance is therefore not a mental state and even less an effort, to avoid generating tension that will quickly give way to fatigue. Practitioners all know people who are in a state of permanent mental alertness and refuse to let go to avoid confronting their inner imbalances, such as those who do not close their eyes during a Shiatsu session, thus preventing the body from speaking. They cover this state with an incessant stream of words. This hyper-control also needs to be dealt with, otherwise the person will exhaust themselves and tense up a little more every day to end up being really sick. True alertness is the absence of mental effort, commonly known as letting go. The state of *zanshin* needs this letting go, to allows attention to be here and everywhere at once, thanks to a continuous presence but without any particular focus. In meditation, this is called full consciousness.

Advantages of zanshin

In Shiatsu, the concept of *zanshin* has two main aspects.

The first is to be attentive to the slightest internal movements of the body (one's own and the recipient's), tensions, pains and temperatures (cold, hot). This also helps to avoid doing any harm by feeling where the limit of pressure is for each individual, to adapt instinctively to a change in the organs or the activity of energy, to accompany the person as accurately as possible and without mishap. Thanks to *zanshin* there are no surprises, just actions and reactions completed in a state of deep tranquillity, which is eminently reassuring for the recipient as for the practitioner.

The second advantage of *zanshin* is the pursuit of intention, even when movement stops. Martial arts practitioners explain this as a technique blocked by immobilization but in which the intention does not stop and continues to flow into the opponent's body. Or as the continuing effects of a blow inside the body, after being given. Or after the end of a technique when the practitioner does not relax but retains a permanent presence, his body and his empty mind already ready for the next step. And all this without physical tension.

Now put all this back into Shiatsu. When the pressure stops, the intention continues its action on an inner journey. This is particularly true during an energy connection between two points. The fact of stopping the mechanical movement does not stop the movement of intention and energy. It is also thanks to this phenomenon that the channels react to the practitioner's ongoing intention. If the points no longer acted as soon as they were released, there would be little or no result. There would be no Shiatsu and only acupuncture would be possible since the needles stay in the same place for a long time. This is the fundamental difference between acupuncture and Shiatsu. With acupuncture, the practitioner offers presence and energy, but only initially. Then, it is the intermediate tool between him and the receiver that continues the work. In Shiatsu, there is no intermediary, and it is an hour of continuous presence, attention and energy that the practitioner must provide, which makes a big difference. As all Shiatsu practitioners are only men and women, they obviously have flaws. And I have frequently had the experience, especially when I started, of starting to think about something else during the session. Very quickly, the receiver returns to the surface of his consciousness, reopens his eyes and sometimes even starts chatting. It then takes a big effort to realize that our attention is no longer there, to go back and to bring the *jusha* back inside himself.

Zanshin expresses itself especially at the end of a session. When contact with the recipient is broken, the effect created by Shiatsu must prolong itself. It is therefore important that the practitioner remains in the state of continuous vigilance until the recipient is gone, in case he needs to ward off an impromptu weakness at the end of the session, for example. This is also a non-verbal message that indicates that the intensity of the treatment is not a temporary passing but a total commitment of the practitioner that will last beyond the hour spent in his company. Traditionally, it is said that the effects of Shiatsu last three days in the Yang phase (with effects that can be felt by the client) which represents the cleansing phase, Then three days in the Yin phase (with subtler effects, more difficult to feel, but just as important for the treatment), which represents the integration phase. It is only on the seventh day that we can treat the person again (unless there is an emergency). During the Yang phase, a meigen[3] (瞑眩) effect can sometimes arise; this is a stronger expression of the symptoms that can look like a worsening of the condition of the recipient. *Zanshin*'s voice is on full display here. Usually after 24 hours (or 72 hours in the strongest cases), the symptoms disappear, as if the body needed to go through a phase of inner crisis to get rid of its blockages and other disorders. It is not for nothing that we talk about an inner journey in Shiatsu rather than healing. As K.G. Dürckheim says: "You have to lose sight of the path once to realize what the path is. We must ultimately lose each other in order to find each other."[4]

Developing attentiveness

As explained above, the continuous presence of the practitioner is the key to the success of a good Shiatsu. If you arrive out of breath, unprepared for a session, the start may be laborious. However, even if you have prepared in advance, you just need to think about something else for *zanshin* to be broken. Indeed, our thoughts form waves that circulate and transmit information. As soon as you think again about your family problems or the shopping list, the receiver will feel the change in the quality of your presence. He can even guess what's going through your mind. But if your mind remains blank, the recipient will feel free to sense and choose his path whilst knowing that he is supported. On the other hand, as soon as the presence of the practitioner decreases, he will feel deserted and will return to the surface of his mind. His mind will wonder what is happening because it will pick up on the absence of the practitioner. This is why a practitioner should never abandon his recipient.

Pedagogically speaking and in order to appreciate how important a Shiatsu principle is, do not hesitate to propose exercises that do exactly the opposite of what we are trying to transmit. Rather than only practising calm, it is interesting to demonstrate that thoughts flow from one person to another. I often play this little game with my students: after a short meditation to calm the mind, I ask them to settle in a circle and we play Chinese whispers but without words. I tell one of them to think very hard about a simple word, a word linked to what we are doing. This word must then be felt by the person. Then, he grabs the inside of the wrist of the person to his right to transmit the vibration, the sensation, and the emotion that this word generated. The recipient does likewise, thus linking the two forearms, and lets himself be won over by the wave emitted by the first. Then without a word, he frees himself and transmits to the next person what he thinks he has understood, and so on until the last person. It is important not to try to analyse what you feel but to make sure to keep only the feeling and the vibration that results from it. For this, the mind must not intervene. I ask the last student who receives the vibration what the word transmitted by the first person was, then I ask the penultimate one and so on until the first recipient. It is striking to note that one time out of three, the last student finds the word and that in almost all cases a person in the circle finds the word or at least its general meaning. By repeating the exercise as many times as there are people in the circle (I recommend not to exceed five or six players), the transmission of thought works better and better.

This little exercise is very informative. The first lesson we can learn is that anyone can receive thoughts and even find the words or their meanings. This makes it possible to understand the need to be calm and free of thoughts when giving Shiatsu. The second lesson is that with an empty mind, one receives the information that emanates from the other. But it is not just the mind that emits waves, vibrations and therefore information. The whole body is capable of this, especially the organs. Therefore, putting oneself in a state of continuous attention thanks to mental Emptiness allows one to receive this information. Finally, and to conclude, the last lesson is that, by repeating the exercise with the same people, more and more often the thoughts emitted are found. In other words, individual energies harmonize to form a group energy. In the therapeutic relationship, the more the recipient returns, the more the *shiatsushi* will be able to deepen his feelings and profoundly perceive from what the recipient suffers.

My mind, seduced and sorrowful,
Has long tried to see
What in your being touches me,
– It's your look, attentive and beautiful.[5]

Summary

1. The term *zanshin* indicates a state of continuous alertness through the abandonment of the mind.
2. Being attentive is not an effort of the mind. In fact, the opposite is true.
3. Mental Emptiness allows the brain to open up and become more receptive.
4. The state of *zanshin* opens up the possibility of feeling everything, but also of continuing an action after the movement ends.
5. There are many exercises to develop the state of alertness/ perception. It is necessary to practise them to realize the importance of a presence without a mind that does not interfere with the technique.

20

Diagnosis Shō

In the thick fog
What does the body cry out
Between hills and valleys?[1]

The full Japanese name for *Shō* is *Shindan hō* (診斷法), meaning "medical examination", because Shiatsu and, before that, Anma are sciences from medical traditions. But within this diagnosis, we only use the four basic steps, because the notions included in this traditional examination are no longer studied today. These were:

- *Ten-Shō* 天象 ("Celestial Phenomena"): how the movements of the Sun, Moon and major constellations affect our health and condition; for example: how a woman's menstrual cycle is impacted by lunar cycles.
- *Chi-Shō* 地象 ("Earthly Phenomena"): how the mountains, the plains, the sea, the desert and the forest affect us all.
- *Ji-Shō* 時象 ("Time Phenomena"): how changes in the seasons and the circadian cycle (alternating day and night) affect us.[2]

Thanks to the attention developed by the practitioner, he will be able to begin to study the Oriental diagnosis known in *Kanpō* (漢方) medicine as *Shō* (証) diagnosis. One could write entire books on the *Shō* diagnosis, which has in fact been the case, especially in Japanese. Before elaborating further, let's clarify some important points. The notion of diagnosis here does not have the same meaning as in Western medicine. Moreover, in Western countries, the term "diagnosis" is reserved by law for the use of doctors only. This is why it is translated as "energy analysis", which by the way reflects much better the reality of what we do in Shiatsu. It should also be remembered that if the Japanese use the term diagnosis, it is also because Shiatsu is recognized as part of the official medicine in the Land of the Rising Sun.

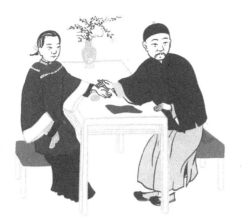

PULSE READING IS THE MOST COMPLEX AND
PROFOUND ART OF ORIENTAL MEDICINE.

Shō is one of the key concepts of *Kanpō* medicine, itself a variant of classical Chinese medicine. The translation of its kanji 証 means "proof".[3] These proofs are in fact the different manifestations of *Ki* that can be found by taking the pulse and observing the face, to name just two examples. As *Ki* is both substance and function, it can be found and deciphered at every level of observation of the body. Every detail of the body and every bodily manifestation is "proof" of whether the energy is working properly or not. In this way, thanks to all the information gathered by the practitioner or traditional doctor, it is possible to establish a precise pathological picture that will pave the way for treatment. Once again, it is important to specify that a pathological picture is not the description of a disease according to the Western conception. The terms used more accurately reflect a situation according to the precepts of Chinese medicine, such as "Lung Heat Invasion" or "Phlegm in the Stomach", which are not the names of Western diseases. What's more, these patterns group together a vast array of symptoms and pathologies, because as always with the ancient Chinese, it is not possible to reduce the various states of health to a single definition. In their mind, this would be too simplistic and would not take into account the permanent inter-actions with the body as a whole and with nature. For example, "Lung Heat Invasion" covers different situations that could be translated as coughing, but it could just as easily be physical agitation, an infection of the respiratory system, asthma, angina, etc. It is then difficult to specify from which part of the body the "Lung Heat Invasion" orig-inates. It is therefore difficult to specify what illness is involved in Western terms, but we can define the quality of the energy (Heat), its state (Empty, Stagnation, Excess) and which organ is affected (in this case the Lung).

The organs of Oriental medicine are themselves different from what we know from scientific anatomy. The lung is an intrathoracic organ that enables vital gas exchanges (enter O_2, exit CO_2), commonly called breathing. On the other hand, the Lung in Oriental medicine is written with a capital letter to avoid confusion between the dif-ferent medical approaches. Here the Lung is not only an organ, it is also much more than that because it represents a set of energetic functions: it ensures the energetic diffusion of protective Ki and Body Fluids,[4] controls the descent of energy in the body, and regulates the internal/external exchanges of individual Ki with that of the environ-ment; it regulates the Water Passages;[5] it controls the surface (skin) and hair system, and finally it houses a part of the human psyche called the corporeal Soul (Po in Chinese). To understand all this, one must obviously immerse oneself in the study of Eastern medicine, but this short list makes it possible to understand once again that the Lung is a rather vast energetic entity and not just an organ.

Once the distinction between Eastern and Western medicine is clearly established, it is then possible to establish the Shō diagnosis, which consists of four phases, or Yonshin Hō 四診法 (literally "the four examinations"), all equally important. These four phases are studied separately mainly for pedagogical reasons. In practice, they regularly overlap. For example, when a person enters a Shiatsu practice, the diagnosis has already started just by observing how the person stands in front of the door. The fact that they shake hands is already part of palpation, whereas the way they walk is part of observation.

As for listening to the tone of their voice, that can be classified as feeling. It is not possible to ask your visitor to separate each aspect so that you can distinguish each Shō, as this would be absurd and very restrictive. This is why the practice of *Shō* diagnosis takes years, or rather decades, before it becomes second nature. Let's now look at the four steps, bearing in mind that it won't be possible here to describe them exhaustively, just to outline their nature.

Observe

Bōshin 望診

This term literally translates as "examination by observation". This term is distinct from the visual diagnosis performed in medicine (called *Shishin* in Japanese). Moreover, the kanji *Bō* 望 means "to see from afar, to see far, far away", which refers us directly to the principle seen in Chapter 18. As for *Shin* 診, this term simply refers to an "examination" (literally "to make it clear"). It is in each of the terms designating the four phases of diagnosis.

This work requires a few years of practice, because it is possible to make a large number of observations in a human being. The first observation that a practitioner must make is how the recipient enters the Shiatsu practice. This already allows you to know a lot about posture defects, body imbalances, muscle tension and joint pain. The observation also concerns the eyes, where the inner Fire or the vital Force of *Ki* is expressed, the light that shines in the pupil – or not, depending on the case. But the eyes reveal a lot more interesting information such as the colour of the sclera, the holes in the iris, veins and venules and their directions, the "sesame seeds"[6] and other aspects. Even richer is the observation of the tongue that indicates the state of a person in this instant. This observation covers colour, shape and lingual coating. There is also a precise mapping of organs on the surface of the tongue, which offers the possibility of "reading" energy imbalances, organ by organ. Note also the colour of the skin, the hair, the map of the nose, face, ears, the position of the feet, toes, wrinkles, and the list keeps going. A lot of details can be observed, and you can spend hours doing it. This is why it is important, in order not to spend too much time on observation, to focus on the details that will confirm or deny the statements of the person.

Although most of the observation is done in silence, i.e., the practitioner does not say what he is observing and noting for himself, this in no way excludes a more active observation. For example, in the case of spinal disorders, don't hesitate to ask the recipient to perform a certain number of well-known movements such as right-left horizontal rotation, right-left tilt, front-back flexion, and to ask the same for the neck. To do this, ask the person to stand up, clearly placing yourself in the position of the close observer. This will enable you to quickly detect the blocking points and deduce the muscular tensions or blockages, and consequently the pain. In this way, you can easily visualize what you need to do during the session to unblock and relieve the pain.

There are also more subtle observations to be made. We have already talked about the *enzan'no metsuke* technique, which allows you to see the whole and not just the details. But it is also possible to observe the language of the body through its movements, nervous gestures or unconscious tremors, particularly those of the hands when the person is speaking. They say a lot about a person's emotional and psychological state. For example, shoulders that are raised, closed and in front of the body are rarely a sign of joy and fulfilment. Quite the contrary! Finally, for those who have developed this ability, particularly through meditation, it is also possible to observe a person's energy field, its thickness, its leaking areas and holes, and for the most gifted, the colours of what is known as the aura.

Question

Monshin 問診

This is an "examination by asking" or "by speaking". Literally, this term has a meaning that speaks volumes: "to verbally question someone about what they hold hidden in their heart." The practitioner asks what symptoms are experienced or observed by the *jusha*. It is important to be aware of cultural factors during this examination. For example, losing face is of great concern to many Japanese people, who will only talk about their physical pain, because to talk about their psycho-emotional pain is to reveal themselves and risk losing face. But talking about one's body is not a problem because, through the ailments of the body, the practitioner will be able to understand what is going on, which avoids what would be embarrassing questions, at least in Japanese culture. In China people are a little less modest and speak more frankly to the one who represents a solution to their suffering, but they will still prefer to talk about the body if they can avoid other subjects. In the West, people tend to talk easily about themselves, their intimate lives, their emotions, which makes it easier for the practitioner to understand. On the other hand, when speech becomes an avalanche of words, it is necessary to know how to regulate and stop this flow, under penalty of spending the session talking without being able to feel what is at stake inside. This is a fairly common unconscious strategy among people who do not wish to confront themselves.

Questioning is itself an art, requiring a good understanding of both what is being asked and what the words prompt in the person. These aspects are very important. If the most obvious question to ask is "How are you?" or "What are your reasons for coming to Shiatsu?", asking questions about health can be much more delicate. For example, anything to do with sex and sexuality can make a person feel embarrassed, as it concerns their intimacy, unless they come specifically for that reason. You should also bear in mind that in all cultures, words carry a symbolic and emotional charge that can be more or less powerful. If you are intrigued by the multiple symptoms presented by someone who is confiding in you and you say to them, "Are you sure you don't have cancer?", it's safe to say that you are going to unleash a wave of potentially devastating emotions. What's more, professionally speaking, you'll have got it all wrong. First, because the disease and its diagnosis are not your responsibility, but that of the oncologists in this case, and second, because you will frighten the person and they will never trust you again. On the other hand, if you ask whether the person is being regularly monitored by a doctor, and whether they are talking to him or her about their various symptoms, this indicates that you are not taking a stand and, better still, that you are perfectly aware of their situation. So, you must choose your words carefully.

The art of questioning requires a good knowledge of a large number of Shō and the pathological patterns to which you might attach to them. For this, it is important to have a kind of tree of questions to ask – as well as all its ramifications – that you would always have in mind. Thus, you can easily leave the common core (everyone has a body, everyone hurts somewhere) to explore the major branches (which represent the major themes), then refine by asking more specific questions as you go. Let's take an example: a person comes because he feels tired and can't get up quickly in the morning. Immediately, the branches of the quiz to explore should light up in your mind.

- **Sleep**: Does the person get enough sleep, when do they go to bed, do they have nightmares, night sweats, do they wake up suddenly?
- **Diet**: Is the person eating enough? What do they eat? In what conditions do they eat?
- **Environment**: Does the person live in a confined space, close to factories or fields sprayed with pesticides? Are they electro-sensitive to telephone or Wi-Fi waves?
- **Relationships**: Are their family relationships good, or is there a conflict that is draining all their energy? Or is it the end of a love story?
- **Work**: Is it physical, intense, unpleasant or boring, or does it involve harassment?
- **Pain**: Is the person in physical pain, in chronic pain, or did they have an accident? If so, in which part of the body? How does it manifest itself? How often does it occur?
- **Illness**: Has the person recently had a check-up to see what is wrong?
- **Psyche**: Does the person feel sad, confined, conflicted, abandoned? Has there been a personal tragedy?

The basic principle of questioning is quite simple: avoid closed questions with a "yes" or "no" answer. They won't get you very far. On the contrary, let the person talk and push them in a direction that allows you to explore the various possible causes of their discomfort. They won't feel constrained by your questions, but on the contrary will feel listened to and will give free rein to what they have to say. For many people, the simple fact of talking already represents the start of treatment and relieves them of a burden. Finally, don't forget to take note of all the information in the answers, so that you can cross-check the ones that come up most often. They will guide you to the organs and channels that are suffering.

An interrogation requires not only knowledge and tact, but also to be a great listener through your presence and kindness. Moreover, both in your remarks and way of listening, I recommend that you use the techniques of non-violent communication (NVC)[7] based on four pillars: observation, feelings, needs, requests. These fundamentals connect us to the notion of empathy, to deep listening, with the ears certainly but also with the belly and the heart. This global listening of the body-mind collects the oral responses of the recipient but also hears/feels all the unspoken. This implies a certain habit of human beings, which requires time, but also listening to one's body. For example, when someone forcefully tells you that the idea you are following on is excluded (sexual abuse for example), do not necessarily throw your idea in your mental trash. A person vehemently stating that this is not the right track does not want you to question further in that direction. Out of respect for the person, do not insist. Yet your intuition, your feeling in the gut tells you that this is where the problem lies. Later during palpation, you will ask silent questions to the body. This is the whole point of the next two steps.

Listen

Bunshin 聞診
These kanji mean "examination by listening to the voice". Here again, the literal meaning is revealing, because *Bun* 聞 means "to seek to hear something indistinct". It is rarely used by Westerners because it is difficult to do, particularly as it does not involve the intellect. The voice carries all the information given by the speech. But its tone, strength and vibration are also waves that carry energy and therefore information other than just words. It's important to feel this energy, because you can hear what's not being said. We also listen for verbal coherence, breathing noises, hiccups, belching, throat clearing, weaknesses in flow or tone. This is why this phase is often more simply translated as "feeling".

Feeling what's in the voice is already a good approach. But more prosaically, you also need to know how to smell the body, which is part of this phase of Oriental diagnosis. Smells reveal a great deal about how well or how poorly the body is functioning. A person with heavy sweating lacks Yin to retain Body Fluids. A person who has bad breath, especially with a rotten egg smell, has a Stomach Stagnation problem. A person who has a pear with caramel smell has a blood disorder that could be reminiscent of diabetes, and so on. Smells of the skin, nose, mouth, hair, feet, sometimes crotch, everything is examined. However, this exercise is by far the most difficult to achieve. Indeed, we have more or less the same smells as our compatriots, simply because we ingest the same foods. In addition to this our hygiene is so important (many people take at least one shower a day, which is catastrophic for the skin and its protection system) that our natural odours are often absent or camouflaged under perfumes. Don't Africans say that Westerners smell like "corpses"?

Ohashi Sensei is by far the most gifted master in this "smell detector" exercise, and he regularly demonstrates this during his courses. He asserts that to succeed in smelling people correctly, you have to radically change your own smell. There are two ways of doing this: move to another continent or change your whole diet. Eating only white rice and vegetables allows you to completely change your smell after several months. Then, the difference between your smell and that of the *jusha* becomes such that its odour will immediately jump out at you. Then all you have to do is learn to identify the cause of the smell.

But smelling is also feeling. The whole body is like an antenna, transmitting and receiving. The more open and sensitive the practitioner becomes, the more he or she will be able to instinctively detect the presence of a problem in the recipient. Here's a case in point: a woman in her forties was complaining of chronic fatigue and a stressful job. But her lower body seemed to be locked in place, vibrating in an unpleasant, chaotic way. Without looking any further, I asked if she'd had a problem or an operation on her lower abdomen. After a long silence, she admitted to me that she had been raped. She hated her whole lower abdomen. This desire to cut herself off from a part of herself was palpable in the air around her and the feeling was able to guide me to the crux of the problem. It's not a magic trick, it's simply a feeling that has been worked on for years. You have to trust yourself and listen to the little voice inside you that guides you to the source of the pain.

Touch

Setsushin 切診

There's a lot to be said about this final stage in the diagnosis. Let's start with semantics. The verb 切 *setsuru* or *kiru*, depending on the pronunciation, literally means "to cut, slice, separate, penetrate, go deep", which may seem rather surprising at first. Indeed, the usual translation of the full term gives us "examination by cutting", whereas we don't do surgery, showing once again in passing that this has nothing to do with modern medicine.

How to understand this term? Here, the hand replaces the blade (in Japanese, they speak of *tegatana* 手刀, or "the hand like a sword"), meaning that it is capable of touching depth. In other words, the practitioner's hand will not stay on the surface as in massage techniques but will find a way to touch beyond the skin, right down to the bone marrow if need be. We understand then that the notion of touch in Shiatsu involves the practitioner far beyond appearances. He must go deep into the tissues and cut the knots that are there. However, if you reread the first chapter of this book, you will remember that you must not force the tissues beyond the point of resistance to avoid too much pain. Some massages (notably Turkish, Thai or Russian) apply pressure with all their might to loosen the muscles. In Shiatsu, this strong pressure is often forbidden (especially in the West, whereas the Japanese like it to remain strong, even painful). The only remaining method is therefore to use the hand as a support, but the intention, presence and attention of the practitioner enable the movement to be extended right to the heart of the pain. The action will then be powerful and gentle at the same time.

In Asia, languages that use characters rather than alphabets like to modify meaning by playing on homophonies. The Japanese are no exception. In this case based on the *"shin"* sound, we can replace the word "examination" with "heart". *Bōshin, monshin, bunshin* and *setsushin* then become "observe with the heart, listen with the heart, feel with the heart, and cut with the heart". This is not an aberration, because in Oriental medicine we learn very early on that the Heart is the house of the Spirit and that it is the only one to feel emotions. What's pleasing about this way of looking at things is that it transforms an examination that might be described as "clinical" into a caring action full of empathy. This is where Shiatsu comes into its own because it acts with the Heart at all the stages we have detailed above.

In the case of *setsushin*, it is a matter of cutting with the Heart, which contains the *Shén* (Spirit), which directs the hand as a bodily extension of the Heart. The mind makes a decision, while the hand cuts into the flesh right where the problem lies. What the *shiatsushi* feels under his hand or fingers is information. Whatever the nature of this information, he feels and acts like a blade to cut away the problem, the knot or the pain. As we have seen from the previous chapters, this treatment is above all an action of the Heart. The Heart, whose noble name in Chinese medicine is "the Emperor", makes it possible to decide (to cut) and give the order to act.

The action of Shiatsu is benevolent, gentle but never soft or indecisive. The practitioner is not a "nice" person, nor one without a big personality. To become a *shiatsushi*, he or she has to show strong willpower and perseverance, confronting himself and then others, overcoming his or her dislikes and fears, touching all kinds of bodies, feeling all kinds of reactions, hearing what he or she doesn't necessarily like to hear. We can draw a parallel here with a doctor, who is confronted with the full variety of human situations. What the Shiatsu Way demands of each student requires a great deal of mental and physical involvement, not to mention changing one's body, one's behaviour, one's lifestyle, one's diet, accepting that one knows nothing, that the receiver is one's master and fighting against an invisible and endless enemy (the pathologies of imbalance). What's more, in order to be available for requests and to be able to listen to the sometimes difficult stories of the people who come to him, he has had to go through many psychological ordeals, cleansing himself internally of his beliefs and fears, so as not to allow the suffering of others to echo within him. This is no mean feat and, in the case of practitioners who have been practising for over 30 years, it can be considered a priesthood. I often find that students who don't make these efforts, who don't try to get out of their comfort zone, sometimes make good technicians if they work regularly, but rarely go beyond that. On the other hand, those who question themselves, meditate, discuss, go back to the books again and again, look within themselves for the reasons for their blockages, those are the ones who are destined for great things.

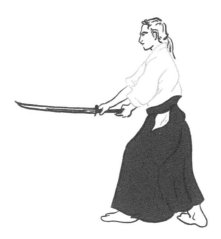

TO CUT INTO THE VOID WITH A SWORD IS TO CUT WITH ONE'S MIND.

Cutting with the hand also means that, with the body as his only tool, he literally cuts through the blockages in the body-mind and cuts through the knots that create imbalances in the recipient's health. To do this, he cannot cheat, he cannot hide behind tools or technology (scanner, ultrasound or MRI) that he could then blame. He can only rely on himself, and the commitment that this requires is a heavy responsibility to bear because he cannot run away from it. We agree that the practitioner does not have an obligation to achieve results, but rather an obligation to use his best endeavours. And this lies in his ability to discern and decide, to make choices. Here again, he can't literally cut up flesh, because he's not a surgeon; and yet that's what he does on an energetic level by using his *Ki* beyond his fingers. He slices through matter, through atoms, through the perverse energy that has settled in, thanks to the vibration of his own energy, which he guides through the recipient.

In martial arts, there are many terms incorporating the word *kiru*. My favourite comes from the world of swordsmanship (Iaido and Kenjutsu): *kiriotoshi*. Literally, it means "to slice, to cut down". The meaning is clearly brutal but above all final. It means the end of the opponent. If we put this term back into Shiatsu, we can catch a glimpse of the "samurai" spirit of the *shiatsushi*, who seeks to cut through the illness once and for all. That said, you need to know how to keep your distance from this samurai spirit, which can turn against you. It's better to know how to cut through and then let go once the person has left the practice. In the world of Shiatsu, there are many cases of practitioners – particularly Japanese practitioners, who are more sensitive to this cultural dimension – who cannot always bear to be held in check by illness. The pathology has to be beaten at all costs, and this becomes an obsession that eats away at them, in turn triggering all sorts of mental, then physical, then physiological rigidities, until they in turn fall ill. Staying with the picture of the warrior, it's best to remember the servant knight of Christianity who kneels and prays over his sword. He relies on Heaven to help him, but he is only an instrument of a greater force. This is exactly what Chinese medicine teaches us. The practitioner is merely the means, the tool through which Yin/Yang, Heaven and Earth, are expressed. *Setsushin* becomes once again the act of cutting, but from the heart with a sword of light and not of steel. It is the righteousness and goodness of the *shiatsushi* that is expressed in this way and not the mind, which changes absolutely everything.

During a discussion in Paris with Ohashi Sensei, I asked him if ancient Japanese martial artists knew how to use the channels and *tsubos*. He replied in the affirmative, that this knowledge was twofold.[8] On the one hand, the points were used to harm and even kill, and on the other, to relax and heal. Obviously, this knowledge was jealously guarded as a secret in the various schools of Budo.[9] But the result was that the warrior or *bushi* who trained to kill or injure quickly found himself confronted with the opposite posture, which was to do good with the same pressure points. For many of them, this forced them to see what they were doing differently. Aided by the Shintō vision, they understood that the world is a balance in perpetual motion and that it is only the intention of the gesture and the mind that can tip the result to one side or another. They could then see that beyond the hands, even the sword (刀 katana) could be used to kill (殺人剣 satsujinken) or to preserve life (活人剣 katsujinken) and protect it.[10] This is *setsushin*: the ability to decide and choose not to harm, but to help, protect and relieve.

Closer to home, and still in the world of martial arts, Shi Dejian is currently one of the great masters of Shaolin Kungfu. Far from the Kungfu business and spectacular demonstrations, his mission is to preserve authentic Kungfu, i.e., Kungfu that does not come from academic training, but springs spontaneously from the body. Living in a remote temple, he has only six disciples. For each of them, the programme is the same and is summed up in his own words: "First, become a good man (meditate, work in the fields, help the community, respect yourself and others). Second, to become a good doctor (herbalism, acupuncture, moxibustion, dietetics). Finally, practise martial arts". It's interesting to hear from a master of this stature the order of priority of these stages, which consists of first acquiring knowledge to heal and then being able to practise martial arts. In the event of injury, the practitioner will be able to heal and repair his mistake.

But what is the use of touch? From the first three steps, the *Shō* diagnosis already gives an interesting energetic assessment. Thanks to questioning, observation and feeling, touch is used to seek confirmation of the evidence already accumulated. Touch is the most delicate and important stage of the assessment. Through touch, we can find - or not - the physical or physiological traces which will determine which organs and channels are affected, and where the Voids, Plenitudes or Stasis of *Ki* are located. Treatment then becomes much easier once this type of work has been carried out. Once again, many palpations are possible. In Japanese culture, palpation of the *hara* is by far the central axis of *setsushin*. The *hara* is the belly, which holds many keys to understanding digestive and emotional knots, but above all it is the seat of the personality. It's not for nothing that only the Japanese invented *seppuku* 切腹, better known as *hara kiri* 腹切り. Warriors chose to kill themselves by cutting open their stomachs. Quite a symbol! As Shiatsu is not a technique of destruction, the *hara* becomes the seat of information and healing, because touching it goes directly to the heart of the person. There are many different ways of touching the belly, far more than can be found on Masunaga's organ map.[11] I encourage the reader to study all the possible styles of Shiatsu to understand the diversity in the treatment of the abdomen.

Another important aspect of palpation is that of the pulse. To be completely accurate, we could talk about palpation of pulses: radial, apical,[12] jugular, ankle, there is no shortage of places. But the radial pulse takes the lion's share, because alone it can provide a wealth of information. Indeed, there are three positions (Inch, Gate, Foot) for taking the radial pulse. These three positions each have three depths (superficial, middle, deep), making nine palpations. As we have two wrists and the right and left wrists do not reflect the same organs, we have 18 palpations to perform. If you add to this the plethora of possible types of pulse (wide, deep, floating, slow, fast, short, long... no less than 26 different types), you'll understand that pulse-taking is an art in itself within *Shō* diagnosis. But by palpating the pulse, you can obtain so much information that some practitioners use this method alone to establish a person's energy balance.

Palpation does not stop at the belly and pulse. As soon as the person arrives, the handshake to say hello is already a palpation. Is the hand firm or soft, cold or hot, calloused or soft, present or absent? How damp is it, what is its texture, is it red, irritated, or cut? This is all information that should not be overlooked. Muscles can also be palpated to determine their flaccidity/tonicity, as they are linked to the sinew channels. You can also use the organ maps on the back, feet, ears and hands to obtain more information. The main meridians are also very useful to palpate, as you can quickly identify where the energy is, where it is blocked and where it is absent. And, of course, we finish by palpating the *tsubos*, particularly those belonging to important families, such as the *Sen* (Well), *Bo* (Gathering), *Yu* (Transport) and other points.

The great characteristic of Shiatsu, and I would go so far as to say its whole secret, consists in palpating and treating at the same time. Masunaga Sensei used to say: "The diagnosis corresponds to the treatment." When the practitioner presses on a *tsubo*, he does two things at once: he questions it (this is palpation in the sense of *Shō* diagnosis) and he treats it (he presses on it to act on it and make it react). This simultaneous dual action is very confusing for beginners, and quite rightly so. In reality, there's a very short time difference between the two actions, but they're really the same gesture. To be clearer, we can say that when the thumb rests on a *tsubo*, it is already questioning it. The beginning of the pressure until resistance is found is still examination by touch. From the moment contact is made with the resistance in the *tsubo*, everything that follows is treatment. But even during this time of treatment, the practitioner continues to listen and to question with intensity everything that is happening in the *tsubo*: variations in energy, rising information, relaxation of the tissues, body noises that accompany the pressure...

At this point, it becomes difficult to distinguish the treatment from the diagnosis, as the two constantly respond to each other. To master this aspect is to master the art of Shiatsu.

Summary

1. The Oriental diagnosis is an energetic assessment of the person. It has nothing to do with Western medicine.
2. *Shō* diagnosis looks for evidence of correct or defective energy activity.
3. *Shō* diagnosis involves four phases: observation, listening, questioning and touch.
4. Touch goes beyond appearances and does not remain on the surface.
5. The art of pressure in Shiatsu lies in the combination of diagnosis and treatment in the same touch.

21

Distances

The human being's usual relationship with the world is based on two fundamental dimensions: space and time. Space designates the directions in which we can move, and time enables us to determine duration (of life, actions, cycles, etc.). Since Einstein, we've known that space and time are in fact a single dimension in which everything is intrinsically linked. But long before the theory of relativity, the Japanese used a term to designate space and time: *Ma-ai* (間合). This term refers to the different distances separating two beings within a meeting.

The distances of Shiatsu

During a Shiatsu session, the distance between the two protagonists varies greatly from moment to moment. At the very beginning, a handshake to say hello formalizes the encounter, establishing a first physical contact and bringing the two people closer together. A respectful distance is then maintained for a while, while the receiver sets down his or her belongings, changes clothes and settles on the tatami or futon. This is the moment for a neutral, informal discussion, respecting the distance that allows the receiver to prepare himself. From the moment the *jusha* is settled in the practice room, the distance shortens. The *shiatsushi* questions, chats, and already observes the eyes, skin tone and many other aspects of the body thanks to this close distance. Then comes palpation, the indispensable phase of Oriental diagnosis. This is when distance is reduced to almost nothing. The practitioner holds himself close to the receiver, to establish a contact that goes beyond the hands alone. He engages his body, and the knees and thighs can easily be brought into contact with the person lying down. Palpation itself is preceded by gentle, non-moving contact. Pressure should never be applied all at once, as this would be too aggressive and risk putting the receiver on alert. On the contrary, the session always begins with a gentle, quiet, motionless contact that already creates an initial bond between the two individuals. During the treatment, the *shiatsushi* moves closer to be as close as possible to the receiver. Then distance changes its nature. With no mental agitation from the practitioner and complete relaxation of the *jusha*, the distance literally melts away. As there can be no closer physical contact, the *Ma-ai* takes place at heart level. The distance here is a movement of the hearts towards each other, to become one, so that the *shiatsushi* can show the way.

To better understand this, we need to decipher the ideogram 間 "*ma*". This is made up of the word for "door" (門, *mon*), going around the character, and within it the radical for "Sun/day" (日, *ri*). In other words, it is daylight glimpsed through the opening of a door. But even a closed door lets in a ray of sunlight through the smallest of gaps. If the receiver is afraid, the door stays closed, and the space seems too small. If he's lost, the space is too big. In other words, he no longer masters distances. The *shiatsushi* guides him gently and with good heart to open the door correctly. But how does he do it? A gap is a powerful force because it contains empty space. Thus, any solid surface that cracks is weakened because the force that unites it is not sufficient to counteract the force of the void. For the distance "*ma*", the gap in the door lets you edge in little by little to open the door, to remove physical, emotional, or psychological blockages. In turn, the character 合 "*ai*" represents union, unity, or literally "those who speak with one mouth under the same roof". The *shiatsushi* therefore unites in a heart-to-heart relationship (以心伝心 "*I shin den shin*") to completely reduce the distance, pass through the gap and open the door to the recipient's heart. It is then that he will see the path to his own healing. We better understand the importance of mental Emptiness. This makes it possible to unite with the void that is in the distance and to achieve a union with the receiver, because the two voids attract each other irresistibly. We also understand that the practitioner is only a trigger and that only the receiver heals himself by accepting – or not – the path opened to him.

Emptiness: The keystone of life

These words may seem obscure to those who do not meditate. In this case, I can only recommend that you get started. But to better understand the concept of *Ma-ai*, we must remember that in our world nothing exists without the void, because it is the Emptiness that gives a purpose. Here is what Laozi says in his *Book of the Way and Virtue*:

> *Thirty spokes around one hub*
> *Employ the nothing inside, and you can use a cart.*
> *Knead the clay to make a pot.*
> *Employ the nothing inside, and you can use a pot.*
> *Cut out doors and windows.*
> *Employ the nothing inside, and you can use a room.*
> *What is achieved is something,*
> *By employing nothing it can be used.*[1]

Take the example of a vase. It is only useful because it is empty and can receive water and flowers. Ditto for the glass, the plate, the bowl and so on. Think of a house. Without Emptiness inside, it is impossible to live there. To bring light in, the walls are hollowed out to create openings, empty spaces that allow light to pass through. A car is only useful because it is empty and allows you to settle in it. The same goes for the vast majority of our objects. If we go down into the infinitely small with the help of an electronic microscope, we see that between the particles of the same atom there is mostly vacuum. And between the atoms, there are more. All matter is made like this, whether it is wood, brick, water or plastic. Even better, we know that this vacuum is the universal glue that allows atoms to stay together. More precisely, it is the electromagnetic forces between the particles that generate the correct distance (space) between atoms. These forces (therefore energy) are the guarantors of the empty space that maintains the cohesion of matter. To summarize, vacuum is the glue that holds matter's shape and prevents dispersion. It's exactly the same thing on a macroscopic scale, otherwise how would planets, stars and galaxies stay in place in relation to each other? Of course, the human being is no exception to this rule. Between all our atoms, we're 99.99 per cent full of empty space. In other words, we're made of little or nothing. As for our digestive tract, it's just a long, empty tube that we regularly fill with food and drink, only to empty again later. Finding the state of Emptiness in this case is a sign of good health. If you stop emptying, you're constipated, and your health will deteriorate rapidly. All our organs and blood vessels are also empty, to enable the transport of blood, nutrients and body fluids. Emptiness is not to be understood here as the absolute absence of matter, but as space in which something can circulate. Students of Chinese medicine are familiar with a space that remains unknown to modern anatomy. Chinese medical texts state that *Qì* circulates in the *Còulǐ* 腠理 space, which lies between the skin and the muscles. The digestive tract also called the *Xūlǐ* 虚理, which is nicknamed the "Hollow Lane" (note the common character between these two terms, *lǐ* 理, meaning "reason, rational"). To conclude once more with meditation, the constantly pursued state of mental Emptiness has a very specific aim: to get in tune with life and become one with the Emptiness that forms the great whole. This is the secret of the famous Yin/Yang symbol.

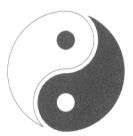

Everyone knows how to interpret the Yin and black side with its little white dot, and conversely the Yang and white side with its little black dot. But how do these complementary opposites hold together? That's the significance of the wavy line that separates the two sides. This line is not a simple line, but the representation of a column of Emptiness that magnetizes the Yin/Yang and holds them together. As in the illustration, simply separate the two parts of the symbol to reveal the Void column.

Ma-ai then changes its meaning. It is no longer simply the distance that separates, but also the distance that enables the two to meet. Let's take martial arts again. In this field, *Ma-ai* is not only the physical space between two opponents, but also the space-time in which the bodies come together to allow the technique to express itself. Without this closeness, the encounter – the fight or the exercise – cannot take place. If there is no encounter, there is no interaction between the two people, and consequently no technique. Distance, a spatial phenomenon that responds to the back-and-forth principles (i.e., Yin and Yang movements) of the universe, thus offers the possibility of creating a space that separates (dilation) followed by a space that brings together (contraction).

Time through distance

Contraction–dilation is the very principle of life, from birth to death. This movement always takes place over a given period of time, be it a few years (human life) or a few billion years (the life of stars or the entire universe). On a smaller scale, this is also what happens in a Shiatsu session. The notion of space is that of the time that separates the beginning and the end of the session, the duration of each phase (welcoming, making contact, energy assessment, treatment, separation), but also the process of self-healing until equilibrium returns to enable good health. As we've already said, you mustn't go too fast or you'll stress the receiver. You mustn't go too slowly either. If you spend 45 minutes of an hour giving a diagnosis, people will get bored and wonder why they're paying you. What they want is something concrete, a solution that works for them, a treatment that provides relief. Time management is also related to rhythm, the time it takes to apply pressure, or the time taken between two pressures. Hand movement is a good example. The movement of the thumbs from one point to another (space) always marks a duration (time). The two concepts are inseparable.

Absence of distance

Problems arise as soon as the distance is not right. In the encounter that is Shiatsu, poor management of the *Ma-ai* can prove disastrous. Imagine opening the door to a client who's coming in for the first time, and then immediately giving them a hug and two sound kisses on the cheeks. What will they think of you? On the other hand, if you don't even shake their hand, you don't smile (distance from the heart), and you stand at a distance from the person without speaking while they settle in, won't they wonder what's going on or what they've done to deserve such an icy welcome? During the treatment, what if you don't touch the person with your whole body, just with your fingertips? Do you really think that the person will come back when they sense a lack of commitment, or even disgust, on your part? *Ma-ai* is not a philosophical idea or an ethereal concept, but a very concrete reality upon which the success of your session and your reputation depend.

In pathology, we often find that it's a lack of space that lies at the root of many symptoms. Commonly, lack of space is what oppresses us the most. Look at people who live in small flats or who are crammed together in an underground train; they say they're suffocating. It's no coincidence that prisoners are locked up in small cells.

It's the same in the body. If there is no more space in the body, the circulation of blood, digestion or fluids is blocked. The blockage will create tension and then pain. Regarding pain, those who suffer physically clearly say that it leaves no respite, offers no space or time in which to recover and regain a little energy. This is a very difficult situation to live with; it can be seen in hospitals all over the world.

Patients want only one thing: for the pain to stop, if only for a little while, so that they can breathe again. The same applies to psychological suffering. Depressive people, for example, are constantly brooding because they no longer have any distance from their negative thoughts. The disappearance of this space should not be taken lightly. An individual who can no longer see in the distance (as in *enzan'no metsuke*) the vast space of the world (physical and psychic) that surrounds him or her faces a real risk of suicide. The absence of space is a terrible suffering, as the poet Louise-Victorine Ackermann puts it:

> *Change your sublime expectations into reality.*
> *But what! to cross them, despite all your impulses,*
> *The distance is too great and the abyss too deep*
> *Between your thoughts and your flanks.*[2]

We've all experienced it when we're under stress: the mind imagines that it no longer has the time to carry out the slightest task, external and internal pressure increases and so does our sense of unease. We know that while stress is not an illness in itself, it is an aggravating factor in the vast majority of illnesses. Once the stressful situation has passed, we find a space where we feel more at ease, where we can express ourselves. This is also true of relationships. If a partner is intrusive, the other quickly suffers and feels oppressed. Conversely, if there is too much distance, worry and anxiety also arise. Whether in the physical body, in our relationships, in our emotions or in our thoughts, *Ma-ai* is the fundamental principle that governs equilibrium. That's why it's vital to know how to recreate space in a person who is suffering, and to take them on a journey into their inner vastness. There are Shiatsu techniques for that.

You're going to think I'm overdoing it, but once again meditation offers a real solution to this problem, because one of the first things we learn to do is to create space between our innermost being (consciousness) and our thoughts (mind) or emotions. With experience, meditators come to realize that time is elastic and that, even in a stressful situation, they have enough space to act or rest. These same exercises also reduce the distance between two people, because in a state of calm, thought waves can be picked up without any magic. In fact, anyone who practises meditation (and we're not talking here about meditation consumed between two breaks and on a smartphone application) will tell you that space and time are altered. You have more time and more space inside to do what you want and think freely. We live at a different pace, as if time has slowed down and the present is stronger. Everything is experienced with greater tranquillity and clarity. In fact, meditation puts the brain on pause and, when it resumes its activity, it is so fit (remember the discussion of potential energy in Chapter 16) that everything seems slow and tranquil. The internal practice of *Ma-ai* thus enables us to distance ourselves from the psychic crises that confine us, to remain mentally healthy and to maintain a permanent state of calm. It is in this space that the relationship is forged, that the *shiatsushi* can act and use the function of the body. More poetically – or more prosaically, as the case may be – we would say that the relationship goes from heart to heart, because it is here that we can reach the Spirit (the *Shén*), through Emptiness.

Summary

1. Respecting physical distances ensures that a session runs smoothly psychologically. These distances vary according to the moment.
2. The term *Ma-ai* implies a physical and temporal distance.
3. In distance, empty space is what allows the separation and attraction of bodies. The Void is therefore the key to relationships, particularly the relationship of matter and the circulation of energy.
4. The absence of physical, psychological or emotional space causes suffering and pain. Putting the body, mind or emotions at the right distance can relieve a person's pain.

22

Linking Energy

The shorter the distance between two people, the stronger the bond. This phase is called *Ki musubi* (氣結び). We've already seen the *Ki* character and its concept of energy, life force, vital breath. The ideogram *Yui*, pronounced *musu* (結), means "to generate, to create, to produce, to engender". In its ancient form, it represented fine silk threads, coiled and knotted together to prevent them from getting tangled. The knot had to be made in such a way as to guarantee the order of the threads and make them strong because they had consolidated. Incidentally, the radical on the left carries in its upper part the meaning "tenuous", and in its lower part the meaning "small". As for the character *bi* (び), here it takes on the meaning of "spirit or power". This word is highly polysemic but is generally translated as "to tie energies", or even more simply "to make the link".

To link the *Ki* between two people is to make the way from body to body, from heart to heart; it is also to link the centres of the three *dān tián* (丹田). These are placed as follows: at the level of the third eye for the *dān tián* of the mind, at the level of the heart for that of the emotions and at the level of the belly for energy. Their connection will enable you to feel spontaneously what is happening in the receiver, or the *shiatsushi*'s intention.

The need for connection

In Japan, the notion of *Ki musubi* is symbolized in the Shintō religion by the creation of enormous ropes. These ropes are laid out in such a way as to connect rocks in the sea, or even islets, to the mainland.

Even though Japan is just a collection of islands, the *Ki musubi* ceremony links all parts of the territory into a single country, which is symbolically very powerful. These ropes can also be seen running across temple frontispieces. It's an expression of the need to unify scattered elements, be they geographical, spiritual or energetic, to give meaning to the whole of nature. This is the etymological meaning of the word "religion", which comes from the Latin *religare*, meaning "to connect". This need to link things - including people - together is a fundamental aspect of the human spirit. We can't conceive of things without meaning, without links, without interactions. Observation of nature tells us that, on the contrary, there are links everywhere. Ecosystems, relationships between people, the mutually engendering cycles of life and death - everything is connected. If nature in all its aspects is interrelated and interdependent, then so must be the human spirit, consciousness and deities. This is the foundation of all religions: to explain the links and make the world coherent.

In the theory known as the Five Movements 五行 (*wǔxíng*),[1] the ancient Chinese noted that there are forces of nature so powerful that they are beyond us. They are both the components and the engines of matter. This observation is shared by all ancient peoples:[2] for the Greeks, Plato cites Air, Water, Earth, Fire and Heaven in the *Timaeus*; for the Celts, Steel, Water, Oak, Fire and Earth; for the Hindus, Solid (*oudana*), Fire (*apana*), Water (*samana*), Life (*prana*) and Air (*vyana*). For the ancient Chinese, these are Water, Fire, Wood, Metal and Earth. When the Earth shakes, when Fire or Water sweeps everything away, we can indeed say that these forces are beyond us. The same applies to the natural creation of ore for Metal and the permanent growth of vegetation for Wood. But Water without Fire makes no sense. It would mean the immediate destruction of the world if only one of these forces existed. Nature exists only because there is a continuous and permanent link between these great powers. Students are familiar with these relationships through the cycles of generation and control. To believe that these two cycles are independent (because they are taught one after the other) is a mistake. It's like having a wheel on one side and bicycle spokes on the other. To move forward, you need the wheel AND the spokes at the same time. The secret of the Five Movements lies in the intimate link between these two cycles. The relationship is as follows: one Element begets another, then one

Element controls another, then begets, then controls and so on. In the end, you'll have gone through the entire cycle of generation AND control in a single movement that retraces both the circle and the five-pointed star.

These notions are covered in detail in Chapter 30.

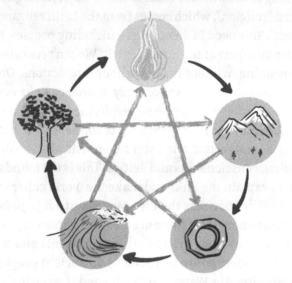

THE SHĒNG 生 GENERATION CYCLE IS ONLY POSSIBLE AT THE SAME TIME AS THE KE 克 CONTROL CYCLE. DELETE ONE OF THE RELATIONSHIPS AND YOU SEVERELY DISORGANIZE THE OTHER.

Connecting in Shiatsu

In Shiatsu, if you leave *tsubos* (points) separated from each other within a meridian (this is the case when there is a Stagnation which forms a dam), the meridian will no longer be perfectly functional. If this disconnection continues over time, increasingly serious symptoms will appear. That's why it's essential to react when the symptoms are at their weakest and above all not to say to yourself "it's nothing serious, it'll go away". Health is something we do for ourselves every day through small, simple but essential gestures: eating healthily and in sufficient quantity, self-massage, resting, revitalizing, using plants, going for walks, enjoying life, and thanking it for its benefits as well as its trials, contemplating, meditating, laughing, playing, etc.

All these little gestures create a long chain of benefits linking your body to your mind, your imbalance to your health. So, it's important to reunite, to connect what's unconnected.

In Aikidō, master Mitsugi Saotome wrote: "In practice, musubi means the ability to harmonise, both physically and mentally, with your partner's energy and movement."[3] Connecting *Ki* means establishing a harmonious link with the other throughout the application of a technique, whether martial or therapeutic. Intention is of course the keystone of this phase. There are two kinds of intention: directed intention and empty intention. Without relaxation and inner calm, the intention cannot be carried out properly. *Ki musubi* can only be achieved if all the concepts discussed above are present. The intention comes from the consciousness (and not from the mind) and simply seeks to make its way through the *jusha's* body to make contact with his energy reserves, Heart and Spirit. Experienced *shiatsushi* say that their fingers feel permanently extended, that they feel at least twice the actual length of their fingers. By dint of practising *Ki musubi*, their physical body lets the energy flow forward and spread all around them (or in the direction of the limbs that are constantly being used, the function making the tool). This is how, in martial arts, the masters feel the attack coming before it starts behind their backs. They are connected to the opponent's intention by their ability to make *Ki musubi*.

In the context of Shiatsu, we would say that *Ki musubi* is the ability to make the link with the *Ki* of the receiver so that we can work together rather than unilaterally. Conversely, if the practitioner believes he knows what is good for the person, he imposes a unilateral point of view, an intention, and an energy without asking the (unconscious) opinion of the receiver. This is a beginner's mistake, but it's not the only one. We often hear practitioners, particularly those who have studied the recipes of Chinese medicine, explain what to do in such and such a case. Kawada Sensei used to say: "There are no recipes in Shiatsu. You always have to adapt to the person." This is true, provided that you also study the pathological patterns of Oriental medicine. These "recipes" are useful, but they must be constantly adapted to the person and the situation. In fact, unlike Western medicine, which identifies a pathology and associates it with a treatment, Chinese pathological patterns are movements, states of imbalance that are constantly fluctuating. This fluctuation makes it possible to create a link between the objective symptoms (which can be observed) and the subjective condition of the person (the psyche, the emotions). This is why a Shiatsu treatment is always personalized. Better still, as the link is re-established each time, the sessions are systematically different, even if it's the same person who comes back week after week.

The energy process

Thanks to *Ki musubi*, the *shiatsushi* will move his energy using his technique and his intention. This is the second possible meaning of *Ki musubi*, as languages that use characters are always polysemous. If you read the kanji differently, you get the following meaning: "the Spirit generates energy". In purely energetic techniques such as Reiki, this process is well explained:

1. The mind creates an intention.
2. The intention is directed towards an area of the body.
3. The energy follows the intention and concentrates in the area.
4. The Blood[4] follows the energy and brings heat and nourishment to the cells; the heat increases the vibration of the cells, dilates, relaxes, and creates a wave.
5. The wave spreads in all directions or, again, follows an intention.

Aware of this process, you'll see that energetics is by no means an obscure, mystical science, but rather child's play. Energetics is a set of mechanisms that respond to relatively simple laws that you just need to know. There's nothing mysterious about it. On the other hand, it can take a long time to get there, as you have to go through all the stages we've seen before, not forgetting a good knowledge of the theories of Oriental medicine if you want to help people.

It all starts with Yin/Yang, the two inseparable energies of Heaven and Earth. If these are indeed two great energies circulating, then the Shiatsu practitioner must be able to connect with them too. This link with heavenly and earthly energy is very important for the *shiatsushi.* By connecting with something greater than himself, he becomes aware of his place in the centre, of his great responsibility as well as his very small person within the universe, which prevents ego from believing itself to be more important than it really is. Once Heaven, Man and Earth are each consciously in their own place, it's time for silence, a silence even more vast than listening to one's own body or that of the receiver. Using intention, we stretch our awareness towards the infinitely high and the infinitely low. A connection then takes place, gently at first, then more rapidly with experience. Heaven and Earth are easy to contact and observe for those who expect nothing. If the intention is to use the two great energies to be stronger, faster, or smarter than others, chances are it won't work well, or for long. Even if you wish to use universal *Ki* to rectify or heal people, this request may still be too egotistical to work. Don't ask for anything, or simply ask for permission to act as a guide to help the person you're treating. We don't heal to shine, nor to have power over others, and even less to be proud of ourselves. We don't actually heal at all. We do our best, with all our heart and with the help of Heaven and Earth, to relieve the suffering of the people who come to us. Yin and Yang are of no particular interest. As the Zen proverb says: "Rain wets everyone, indifferently." The same goes for the two great energies that bring their strength to all that lives and vibrates, without distinction. Once the intention has been set, the practitioner will feel the connection taking place within him. He'll be able to draw on his own energy and on the infinite reservoirs of Heaven and Earth, which is far less tiring and means he can go on for long days without burning out. All that's left to do is to let them flow through the body and guide them to the arms, then through the hands.

Of course, we are first and foremost terrestrial beings, so the Earth's influence is the strongest. In fact, we drink the Earth's water, eat its plants and animals, and breathe its air. The Moon is a detached piece of Earth, which is why it is one of the Yin forces because it is a detached piece of Earth, and that it also generates tides and women's menstruation. Although Yin's presence may be more subtle, softer, and therefore less immediately perceptible, on our human scale it is the most constant and pervasive. Thus, we can easily count on it. Heaven brings its Yang touch, which creates and maintains the movement of life. On our scale, Heaven can seem more fickle despite its power, like the Sun playing with the clouds. It moves fast and strong. Of course, these are only images, as the reality of Yin/Yang is indescribable. This doesn't mean you can't feel them at all times. The quality of their presence is proportional to the quality of the vessel that receives them, i.e., to the quality of what we are.

Summary

1. Linking people, the elements of nature and concepts is a fundamental principle of the human mind. It is this need for coherence that enables us to understand the world and generates the rise of religions.
2. *Ki musubi* is about connecting the energy of the body and the universe.
3. Connecting with the receiver is an essential step in Shiatsu, otherwise you will not feel anything.
4. To perform *Ki musubi*, you need to understand the basic process of the energy arts.
5. The link with Heaven and Earth allows the practitioner to get less tired in his treatments, whilst respecting Yin/Yang.

23

Letting the Energy Flow

Following the logic of the stages step by step, the concepts unfold one after the other. It is not always easy to understand them, let alone feel them. But not knowing them is like walking in the dark without knowing that lanterns exist and that they can light your way. The masters of ancient Asia have been thinking about all this for a long time, so why reinvent the wheel? Let me remind you that master, teacher or senseï (先生) means the one who was born before.[1] Let's follow their example, as Laozi so aptly reminds us: "Experience is a light that only illuminates the path travelled."[2] So let us follow the path set by the masters of the past.

From Ki musubi to Ki no nagare

Once *Ki musubi* has been achieved, the *shiatsushi* can intercede with the *Ki* of the receiver. Remember that without the step of creating the energy link, only the practitioner's *Ki* intervenes; in other words, the practitioner uses his or her own energy to change the state of the receiver. In this game, the practitioner will quickly become drained and tired, and will eventually fall sick in turn. Of course, he can connect to Heaven and Earth to benefit from an additional energy supply which will make him less tired, but it will always pass through him. What is more, it's a disservice to the person coming for treatment if they learn nothing during the session. The practitioner's presence and his or her ability to use his or her inner resources is a teaching that the recipient's body receives. When we say "to heal oneself" we need to understand that it is the receiver who is seeking to heal himself and not the practitioner who is healing. Rather, I would say that the practitioner educates the receiver to use his own resources. If this is not the case, the practitioner and Shiatsu are only crutches that the person cannot do without. It is essential to teach them to walk on their own.

This is the stage of *Ki no nagare* (気の流れ), which contains several meanings at the same time. First, *nagare* (流れ) contains the idea of flow, while the character *no* stipulates the possessive in relation to what is placed before it. This is easily translated as the "flow of *Ki*". In other words, the energy will be like a river, free to flow powerfully and naturally. In fact, in the ancient form of the character, there was the radical of water twice, with a woman in the centre giving birth to a baby head downwards, in the best possible conditions. The notion of flow was an echo of Taoist thought (cited in the works of Laozi and Zhuangzi) which stated that the infant has the characteristics desired by the Way (道 Dào). He has no internal duality, and his gestures are natural and fluid, yet efficient. In other words, he acts naturally because he does not know any conflict.

The notion of flow is particularly relevant in Shiatsu. Without this flow, the *Ki* cannot allow Yin/Yang to circulate, transport Blood and enable the necessary transformations (of food, for example) for our biology to function properly. Flow is life itself, and vice versa. Oriental medicine often compares *Ki* to a stream of water. If the water flows freely, it is clear and joyful, and life proliferates everywhere it comes into contact with. Block it with a dam and the water stagnates, turns green, loses oxygen and ends up rotting. Vegetation regresses and rots too. Flow is therefore fundamental to our health, both physically and psychologically. If a person becomes fixated on the fear of losing something, they will tend to freeze up and want to control their entire environment, their family, their actions, and their emotions. They quickly become manic, bitter, worried, and live in fear of things changing. On the other hand, accepting that everything is only change allows thoughts and emotions to flow freely. In Oriental medicine, the *Ki* of the Heart and Brain is said to circulate freely[3]. In Qìgōng, the great teacher Bruno Lazzari says that "running water never goes stale". Incidentally, here's another Qìgōng adage that may be useful to you:

导气令和, 引体令柔 (*Dǎo qi ling hé, yǐn tǐ ling róu*):

Guiding the *Qì* to create harmony, directing the body (in the sense of training it) to make it soft (or supple, depending on the context).

In other words, by training the body to be soft or supple, it is possible to guide the energy to harmonize the interior, whether for yourself or another person. Once again, nothing should be forced, either physically, intentionally or energetically – this is the key to success. Generally speaking, not imposing implies that the receiver cannot fight and block the technique because nobody is attacking him or her. As O Sensei Ueshiba said: "Nobody can defeat me because I'm not there."

During meditation classes, the theme of blocking, particularly psychological blocking, often comes up. I explain that trying to block the movement of life – which is constantly changing – is an illusion. Anyone who does so is in for a serious disappointment. Whether we like it or not, nature follows the changes of the seasons, the years go by, and time passes. We age little by little, and there's no point in applying anti-wrinkle creams to give ourselves the illusion that this won't happen to us. Movement is like water in a stream tumbling down the slopes to reach the sea. Nothing can stop it. If you go on holiday to a beautiful spot in the countryside, try this experiment: stand in a stream or river and try to block the current with your arms. Not only will this not work, but you'll soon feel your muscles tense up. All you'll get is a cramp. It's the same with our mind, our ideas, our beliefs and our physiological processes. The slightest blockage makes us tired, which is why tiredness is always the first sign of an imbalance, a signal that should not be ignored, let alone deliberately ignored. So, as the Buddhists say: "The only permanence is impermanence." We have to be willing to let go of what we have inside and outside ourselves. Better still, it's better to go with the flow. To quote the *Yi Jīng*: "The only thing that will never change is that everything changes all the time."[4]

The flow of Ki in Shiatsu

Letting energy flow is good, but supporting it is even better. To use the example of the river, swimming against the current just wears you out unnecessarily. It's better to go with the flow. This is the art of the practitioner. When we come across an energy blockage or a muscular knot, there's no point in fighting the problem with all your might. This way of acting runs the risk of creating a myotatic reflex[5] or psychological tension. Bear in mind that at the slightest warning – in other words, at the slightest pain – the receiver will lose confidence in you and won't come back to see you. On the contrary, it's better to increase the amount of energy flowing through the meridian before and after the blockage. It's like a dam of leaves and branches on a stream. If the flow increases, the dam is washed away. Once again, flow is not only desirable but is often the solution to the problem.

In the relationship between the *shiatsushi* and the receiver, *Ki no nagare* also takes on its second meaning, which is "to guide". Thanks to the *Ki musubi* that has formed an "energy knot" between the *shiatsushi* and the *jusha*, the practitioner will literally guide the recipient's *Ki* through his or her body to regulate it and allow it to flow correctly. In this way, the recipient learns (albeit unconsciously) to heal himself. This is the path to healthy self-sufficiency. In other words, thanks to the practitioner's guidance, *Ki no nagare* can trigger the self-healing forces present in each of us. Anatomists will speak of reactivating the parasympathetic nervous system, while energy specialists will speak of restarting and balancing energies. Words don't matter, only the result. Given that *shiatsushi* can only accompany the recipient for a limited time (1 to 2 hours a week at best), the receiver's *Ki* must be trained to repair the dysfunctions of the body and psyche. In this way, they will get into the habit of correcting themselves and will be able to do so on their own after a while. The receiver can then stand on his own two feet.

The question arises again of how to do this. The previous chapters have partially answered this question with the notion of Emptiness, neutral intention and openness of spaces. But the practitioner must also know how to guide the flow of *Ki*. Two parts must be distinguished. First of all, the practitioner will seek to stretch upwards on the one side, to Heaven, and on the other side downwards, to Earth. Preparation before a session is of the utmost importance here. Thanks to this inner tension with which the practitioner is at one (intention can be read as "Un-tension", i.e., a link with Unity), he or she will create a presence beyond the physical body. Along this presence, which is like a straight thread, Yin and Yang will cling and then follow the thread to the practitioner. The two energies will then pass through the practitioner's body with greater force than usual, if the practitioner's body-mind does not create any disturbances in the process. All you have to do is let these two energies mix at the level of your heart and let them flow through your arms, hands and finally your fingers. In this way, the practitioner no longer empties himself, since he is drawing from the endless, bottomless reservoir of celestial and terrestrial energy. This connection is felt particularly in the spine, sometimes signalled by a little inner shiver, then the Three Burners rise in heat, quickly followed by the *Rōkyū* (勞宮 "Palace of Work") points in the centre of the hand, on the Pericardium channel.

Once the practitioner has been able to capture this immense energy and guide it through his hands, he must still let it flow into the body of the recipient. Thanks to *Ki musubi*, the relationship of trust is installed, which facilitates the work. *Ki* will follow this link from heart to heart. However, sometimes the practitioner must move from a neutral intention to an active intention. To do this, he will visualize the area to which he sends the energy, follows its path and observe if the desired action happens. This intention is not a thought or action programmed by the brain. It's more of a half-thought, half-emotion form. Furthermore, you must not want to send it as an object (like a tennis ball) but rather offer it as a gift. The energetic charge of this intention will be better received and will better benefit the receiver, who then has the choice to accept it or not.

Knowing how to guide energy

Of course, you can't learn to guide energy by reading a book. It's a more or less lengthy process that every aspiring *shiatsushi* has to go through, even if some have undeniable gifts. To learn how to act correctly, you need to work hard, repeat yourself and receive guidance from a master. Learning energetics can only be done in a relationship of trust between master and student. Having said that, it is possible to develop a large number of exercises that have a rapid effect. The teacher will take great care to give the exercise without ever influencing or judging the students' feelings. The best thing to do is to divide the class in two and give the instructions to the givers without the receivers hearing anything. Their feedback after the exercise will be all the more interesting as they were never aware of what was going on.

To teach *Ki no nagare*, you need to make regular connections, first without intention, and later with the correct intention. The deeper the connection, the greater the student's ability to reach that depth. In the beginning, it's enough to let the energy circulate between one hand and the body of the receiver. A little later, a two-handed connection can be made. The practitioner's *Ki* will always seek to link the hands together; it's almost automatic. It may take some time at first, but you'll always get there in the end. Gradually you can make the exercise more difficult by doing the same thing but choosing a movement between the two hands (a spiral, for example). When the receiver indicates that they feel a circular movement inside them, it's a winner.

You can also guide the energy to make a detour to an area that is not directly between the two hands. For example, place one hand on the belly below the navel and the other in the small of the back. But instead of letting the energy flow naturally along the shortest route, direct it towards the stomach before reaching the other hand. The hands are located here on very important energetic zones (CV 6 *Kikai* and GV 4 *Meimon*) and this energy will strengthen the stomach. As the receiver knows nothing about the exercise, we simply ask them to comment on how they feel. When they identify a sensation of presence, connection or any other stimulation in the stomach, this means that the goal has been reached and that the exercise can be stopped.

Another more advanced exercise involves grasping both ankles and connecting to the tibia bone, which lies not far below the flesh. The aim is to move down into the marrow and then slowly back up along the bone structure, working your way through the entire skeleton. When you think you have reached the top of the skull, gently release the pressure and once again ask the co-student how he feels. With practice, active intention is less and less necessary, and the advanced practitioner will let the *Ki* flow where the recipient's body calls for and attracts the energy, i.e., where it is needed.

I particularly like the next two exercises, because they always give very clear results.

The first involves making contact with a Source point, such as KD 3 (*Tai'en*). The giver's task is to gently move through the entire Kidney meridian. Not only will the *jusha* say that he feels that "something" is moving up his meridian (or that he senses a progressive filling at work), but the giver will also sense from a distance the blocked areas in the channel and feel the barriers that need to be lifted. It's a very useful exercise which doesn't require any great knowledge, apart from "seeing from the inside" (feeling) the path of the channel.

The second exercise is the use of the Five Movements. These primordial Elements are very powerful, so it's important to prepare the donors well and first tell them to evoke a gentle image linked to one of these Elements. For example, if one of them chooses Fire, suggest a roaring fire in the fireplace on a winter's evening rather than a forest fire. Then the student should put this image in their chest and feel it with all their heart. Then he connects to the channel of his choice and moves up it with the gentle intention of the Element within him. Once the exercise is over – which should take at least ten minutes – ask the receivers to say what they felt, as they still don't know anything. What they say is astonishing. The Element has generally been successfully transmitted and will strengthen the individual.

Summary

1. *Ki no nagare* means the flow of energy and implies a free mind, empty of all thought and a connection to the *Ki* of the receiver.
2. *Ki* flows like water and the practitioner's presence without intention will reinforce its flow.
3. In certain cases, the practitioner guides the flow of *Ki* to obtain certain effects, but this requires practice.
4. Guiding *Ki* can be learned. Many exercises are possible, from the simple connection to the unblocking of a meridian from a single point.

24

Meeting and Harmonization

*D*e-ai (出会) simply means "meeting". But by deciphering the kanji, the term takes on a whole new dimension. The kanji *shutsu* (出) means "outside, exit" and by extension "to go out"; as for the kanji "*ai*" (会), it means "meeting, association, union". So, we end up with a semantic translation that could be "to go out to meet".

We can consider this meeting right from the start, when we open the door, shake hands, make first contact and even throughout the session. A Shiatsu session is a manual treatment and, at the same time, much more than that. The encounter takes place on several levels (physical, emotional, psychic, energetic and even symbolic) and we can communicate with the recipient on several levels. Humans being what they are – complex – there is no lack of levels and layers, so the encounter is not something rare or extraordinary. But for the *shiatsushi* and the *jusha* to meet, at least one of them must leave home. Better still, for the receiver to unite his body-mind, he needs to step outside himself, outside his immediate consciousness, to go beyond his mind. This is the hidden meaning of *De-ai* in Shiatsu.

Silent meeting

However, when the *shiatsushi* makes a connection between two points on a meridian or two areas of the body, he does not necessarily choose to send "only" energy where there is a lack. He can also simply come into contact by reducing the distance (*Ma-ai*) as much as possible.

At this point, the two protagonists feel a connection that goes beyond simple touch.

When the practitioner has crossed the superficial *Luò*, the main channels, the deep *Luò*, the membranes, the Extraordinary Vessels and even the bones, what does he find under his fingers? When he gradually penetrates a *tsubo* and crosses the different layers that make it up, what does he come into contact with? In Shiatsu, this question always remains unanswered because it leaves the technical path for the mystical path belonging to the world of spirituality. Everyone will find their own explanation, depending on their culture and how far they have progressed along their own path. Whatever the case, this is a very profound encounter that surprises and shakes things up. Why is this so? Because this encounter is a two-way street.

Until now, only the practitioner has acted, guided, and educated the recipient's body-mind. Even in the moments of *Ki musubi* and *Ki no nagare*, it is still he who is in control, so to speak. But when this type of encounter occurs, it is the depth of two beings that comes into play. This depth is not mental since thought has already been put on hold in the previous stages. This encounter is not intentional either, because we are not looking for anything. It just is. I'll quote Bernard Bouheret again on this question: "When you get this far into the body, you're no longer in the body. We encounter the indescribable nature of the being, its foundation, its timeless consciousness."[1] A lovely phrase, but one that remains incomprehensible until you have actually experienced this state, which is by its very nature indescribable...

One day in May, a Belgian woman in her late forties came to the practice, complaining of sleep problems and anxiety. I looked for clues using all the tools at my disposal but found nothing conclusive. I began to work on her stomach to unblock it and, once this was done, I placed one hand on her *hara* and the other on the top of her skull. After a while, images of eagles, endless plains, snow and horses come to me. I felt her tense up and then literally start to "light up the room" with the intensity of her vibrations. The energy crackled under my hands. We stayed like this for a while until a deep relaxation came over her body. At the end of the session, I said to her: "If I say the word Mongolia to you, what does that make you think of?" Stunned, the woman told me that only the day before she'd been looking at pictures of the country on the Internet and that she'd been dreaming of going there ever since she was a little girl. "Have you already planned your holiday?" "No," she replied. "So, take a flight to Mongolia this summer and don't plan anything in particular. Let yourself be carried along by the people you meet." This woman did not come back for another session. In fact, she didn't come back at all and, a year later, I received an email telling me that she was taking a shamanism course and thanking me for having been able to "read her soul", saying that she was writing this message because her guide had asked her to thank the person who had pushed her to come all the way here. These are her own words. This is an example of a silent encounter in the depths of the individual. In reality, there was no "soul reading" or anything of the sort, they were just words. On the other hand, there was an exchange of information between our two minds via the circulation of energy.

When this situation arises, there are two options open to us (always that famous free will of ours). Either we accept this encounter, or we refuse it. There is no right or wrong in this, just choices that are not ours to make. When two beings are not compatible, it is better to return to less profound levels to continue the Shiatsu session without disturbing either person. In the feedback from students, it regularly happens that they feel rejected by a particular point or anatomical area. The most sensitive ones quickly withdraw their hands and continue elsewhere. They instinctively sense that they are not welcome, and that the receiver is not ready to open up, at least not yet. It's important not to force the issue, as this can lead to situations that are difficult to manage. The body-mind has its own logic, and this must be respected if the session is to run smoothly. To put it simply, if the meeting is refused, don't make a mountain out of a molehill. It's just that it isn't meant to be. Remember that the *shiatsushi* is not a superman or superwoman, but simply a man or woman who has worked hard to get where he or she is.

In the martial arts, the concept of meeting has two levels. In training, particularly with weapons, the aim is to work in harmony as a pair, to be synchronous. The term *De-ai* is then used in confrontation. This level is considered to be the absolute mastery of *Ma-ai* (timing and distance), because *De-ai* and *Ma-ai* are intrinsically linked. It allows you to understand and feel the moment when the movement is going to start, avoiding any rush or unpleasant surprises. To carry out this principle, you need to achieve total physical availability and a mental Emptiness that excludes any inattention. Vigilance and inner calm are fully deployed. Then time becomes elastic, and you can move without fear within the encounter. If you put this principle of encounter into Shiatsu, you will not only be in silent communication with the *jusha*, but you will also be in such a state of attention that nothing will surprise you and you will instinctively know when to act and when to wait. To paraphrase the masters of meditation, you'll be living in the here and now.

Union in the encounter

When the door to the depths opens, we reach the state of *awase* (合わせ). This term covers a whole host of meanings: "unity, harmonization, coming together, combining, connecting", but also "facing each other, opposing" in Japanese. Let's go back to the martial arts perspective. *Awase* is the marvellous moment when two opponents at odds with each other experience a moment of grace, one might even say beauty, in which opposition no longer exists. They progress together through a technique to its end. But the end comes suddenly, and the two fighters are separated, either by the death of one of them, or by physical submission, which is generally painful. The break is complete, and the whole operation lasts no more than a few seconds.

Shiatsu is different, because the *shiatsushi* does not fight against the receiver. He seeks to rebuild, rebalance and re-harmonize him with his own nature. And to achieve this, he takes his time. In this context, if *awase* is achieved and the two beings merge, amazing results, that some would describe as miraculous, can be obtained! *Awase* is the supreme concept of Japanese arts and techniques. It's a bit like this poem by Kobayashi Issa:

> *An enormous frog and I*
> *Watching each other,*
> *Neither of us moves.*
> *It is unity in the silent encounter.*[2]

However, Shiatsu masters who have a good 30 years' practice behind them can achieve this state without too much energetic risk. Their experience is vast, and they can move confidently forward in this union between two beings. This is particularly useful when they are seeking to undo serious life-threatening imbalances, or in what I call "diseases of the soul".[3] But to achieve this state, you need to have a very strong anchor, to be able to achieve unity without losing yourself in it, in other words, to be able to remain a guide and not "fly away" in this experience. This is a very specific domain area and, generally speaking, Shiatsu schools do not teach techniques or talk about it. On the other hand, the meditation masters I've met around the world are relatively familiar with this state. With a simple touch of their hands, they know how to take a person beyond themselves and live the experience with them. But without going that far, each of us can still do a lot. Just think about one thing: the inner space you create during meditation will automatically include your receiver within you, and therefore allow you to go out and meet him or her during a Shiatsu treatment. The greater your inner space, the more you will allow the person to encounter his or her own depth.

Summary

1. The encounter (*De-ai*) is the moment when the practitioner has complete control over timing and distance.
2. *De-ai* requires unfailing, stress-free attention.
3. *De-ai* allows the practitioner to ensure that everything runs smoothly and with peace of mind.
4. If the encounter leads to unity (*awase*) between the two people, know how to welcome it and remain cautious if you are not advanced on the Way.
5. Here, non-intention seems to be the best way of approaching the person.
6. Thanks to meditation, the encounter is fully welcomed. Meditate to remain stable, to keep your feet on the ground and your Heart in Heaven.

25

The Hand Takes Precedence

When a person entrusts his body and his problems to a Shiatsu practitioner, he is in a situation of demand. This request triggers a whole series of actions by the *shiatsushi*, the aim of which is to relieve the individual while remaining within the professional framework of his or her technique.

The practitioner's main tools are his or her hands. It's obvious, but sometimes it's worth the reminder. Every time the recipient's body changes (physically or emotionally), the *shiatsushi* feels the internal movements of energy in his fingers and reacts accordingly.

He doesn't think, he doesn't interpret (at least not during the treatment phase; the thinking is upstream, during the four phases of the *Shō* diagnosis). He feels and lets his hands come and go on the person like a pianist who knows his score but also knows how to improvise when necessary. But what does this mean? Does it mean that every time the body reacts, there must be a counter-reaction to calm the person down? The answer can be found in the words of the founder of Aikidō, O Sensei Morihei Ueshiba. During an interview in 1957,[1] he was asked whether it was necessary to react to any attack with a defence and gave this response:

> Not at all. It's not a question of timing and speed when responding to an attack. If I had to put it into words, I'd say that you control your opponent without trying to control him. This is the state of constant victory. It's not a question of winning or losing against an opponent.

In this sense, there is no fight in Aikidō. Even if you have an opponent, he becomes a part of you and becomes a partner.

I like to think that the same is true of Shiatsu.

Before the hand

Sente 先手

In Japanese, the kanji *sen* is also read as *saki* and can be translated as "before" or "in front of", depending on the context. The term is regularly used in Japanese martial arts in expressions such as "*go no sen, sen no sen*" or "*sen sen no sen*". But in this sense, *sen* is an abbreviation of the word *sente*, which means "initiative" or "direct". The word *te* means "hand", as in Karate (空手).[2] In other words, it's about letting the hand take the initiative and direct the process without involving the mind or the rational. This way of acting is a high form of Shiatsu that can be found in the principles of Seiki (整気).[3] This technique is a spontaneous and purely energetic form of Shiatsu which has no preconceived scheme for the use of the hands, or points to press on. The idea is to let them follow the natural movement of the *Ki*, to let them move over the body, without trying to impose any kind of vision and even less to try to understand what they are doing. The letting go is total in this case. This minimum work is directly in line with the Chinese Taoist notion of *Wú wéi* or "non-acting". Non-action does not mean that the individual does nothing, but that he or she is not at the origin of the movement, the intention or the action. He accepts that it is nature that makes the decisions, and the practitioner simply follows this path.

This is exactly meaning of the term *sente*; it can also be translated as "before the hand". Before the hand acts, the body feels and accepts, even if nothing visible is happening. The practitioner reacts to this feeling by letting himself be guided and not by applying his will. This happens all the time in everyday life. You have a premonition, an intuition strikes your mind, you sense a situation from a distance. In all cases your body picks up on it and reacts before you even realize it. You then choose whether or not to follow your instincts – it is a question of choice, and therefore of individual freedom. If you listen to your intuition, you'll be surprised to discover that your reaction was perfectly in sync with events. If you don't, you usually learn a little later that you had the right intuition but didn't follow it, which is just as surprising and gives you food for thought for the next time.

Pre-consciousness of the body

But how can we explain the fact that there is a thought that precedes our own thought, or rather an intention that precedes our brain?

In meditation, this notion is linked to the individual's personal unconscious, which is connected to the collective unconscious of all thinking beings. Meditators, even beginners, often have this experience: as soon as their mind becomes calm and no longer agitated in all directions, the conscience[4] receives auditory or visual messages or spontaneous thoughts (we know that we know but we don't know how). With experience, it is quite possible to maintain an active dialogue with your conscience, to ask questions and obtain answers (even if these are not always pleasant to hear). It happens to everyone. All you have to do is look for information in your head and then you can't find it. Or you're working on a maths problem and no solution comes to mind. Then you move on to something else or go to sleep and, after a while, the answer comes. If it was forgotten information, it concerns the individual unconscious. If, on the other hand, it is a solution to a previously unknown problem, your conscience has tapped into the collective unconscious.[5] In fact, at least once in your life, you will have noticed that inventions, scientific discoveries or even your own ideas arise in several people around the world at the same time. This shows once again that we are all connected.[6]

In Chinese medicine, this notion of pre-existence "before the hand" is linked to the notion of Shén, or "Spirit" in the broadest sense of the term. Shén is conceived as the separation of a small part of Heaven (known as the Pre-Heaven Essence), the immense unity that dominates us, and seeks to become incarnate.[7] By choosing incarnation, the Shén experiences matter and divides itself into several visceral entities called the "organ spirits". There are five of these (Po of the Lung, Hún of the Liver, Yi of the Spleen, Zhi of the Kidney, and Shén of the Heart). To make things simple, the Shén is located in the

Heart, works in the Brain and is expressed in the intensity of the eye's pupil. This means that the human being is both a being of flesh and bone (materiality of the post-Heaven Qì) and a spiritual being (immateriality of the Pre-Heaven Essence). Hence the difficulty in finding a balance in this earthly life between material desires and spiritual desires. We are perfectly capable of living on a purely material level, in our own bodies, as well as elevating ourselves and communicating with the spiritual, since it is within us. The *Shén* has the ability to connect with the Pre-Heaven Essence – if we give it the chance – and thus to give our actions the right direction. The advantage of proceeding this way is that we no longer need to use our mind, to try to control, structure, organize... The practitioner who follows this *Wú wéi* path is always free and sure of doing the correct thing.

A story of hands above all

You don't need to be a genius to understand that the first medical tool available to Man was his own hand. He had his hands with him long before he started inventing objects. But apart from that, it is interesting to reread the *Huángdi Neijīng* once again. In Chapter 12, it describes the specific treatments from different regions of China according to climate. Qi Bai describes that in the East, stone chisels are used; in the West, drugs are used; in the North, moxas are used; in the South, needles are used. For a Westerner stopping here, nothing seems shocking and everything seems in order, since we have just covered the four cardinal directions. For an ancient Chinese, however, the fifth direction – the centre – is missing. This is why Qi Bai goes on to say that the treatment at the Centre is massage, mobilization and gymnastics.

The notion of the Centre in the Asian mind is fundamental. The Centre is the place of departure and arrival, the place around which the other directions will revolve. To put something at the centre is to insist on its importance and primacy. To say that at the Centre, the treatment is massage, mobilization and gymnastics is to say that working with the hands and the body is the most important medical art, the first and the one on which all the others depend. What does a doctor do when someone says they have a pain in a particular part of the body? He palpates it. What does an acupuncturist do to locate the precise spot to insert his needle? He touches it with his fingertips. What does a surgeon do before cutting into flesh? He feels around and checks that there's nothing to stop him cutting.

This is why the hand comes first.

And now, how do you rehabilitate a person? By teaching them mobilization exercises. How do you strengthen their body? By encouraging them to do sport. How do you correct structural defects? By showing them how to work on their posture.

How do we maintain our health? By practising gymnastics, stretching and mobilization as long as possible. That's why the body comes first.

The hands' memory

For some years now, scientists have been aware of the importance of our belly,[8] of the digestive system in particular, on our psychological and hormonal life and, more particularly, on our daily well-being. Better still, it has been discovered that this "second brain" has as many neurons as a dog's brain. It is a long way from the main brain, but surprisingly important for a physiological system. Think for a minute about all that a dog is capable of achieving and learning, and you'll understand that the belly is capable of storing a huge amount of information.

What about our hands? For the moment, no scientific study has been conducted into the potential memory of the hands. However, it has to be said that they have their own intelligence. We already know that blind people can feel the heat of a colour and guess the colour quite accurately, which says a lot about the sensitivity of skin sensors. But over the years and dozens of discussions with my colleagues, we've all agreed on one thing: when we no longer know who we're dealing with from one session to the next, all we need to do is put our hands on the body and everything quickly comes back to consciousness. Do this test if you're already a little advanced in Shiatsu: don't prepare for your session with someone you've already had. Make sure that the patient's name means nothing to you and that you have forgotten everything about the previous session. Welcome them as usual, without any fear, and then place your hands on their stomach. You'll see that the memories come flooding back: why the patient came in the first place, what you did last time and what treatment to carry out now. It's astonishing!

So, I claim – without any scientific proof – that the hands retain the memory of what they do.

Summary

1. The hand is the ultimate tool of the Shiatsu practitioner and of human in general.
2. Intention precedes the hand, a concept called *sente* in Japanese.
3. The hands follow their own logic and memorize the information received from the receiver's body.

26

The Heart

Let nothing belong to me.
Only the peace of the heart
And the freshness of the air.

KOBAYASHI ISSA[1]

Like a backdrop that lies behind all the notions we've covered so far, the Heart returns regularly as both the starting point and the end point of everything we do in Shiatsu. The kanji 心 *Kokoro*, also read *Shin*, has several meanings at once: the heart as an organ, the cardiac muscle that pumps blood; the Heart as the home of the Spirit and the emotional centre of the individual. The Spirit character 神 (*kami*) is pronounced *shin* in Japanese, in near homophony with the Chinese word *Xin* (the heart again, pronounced *sin*), because Japanese culture grew out of the study of Chinese language and philosophy, before setting itself apart and finding its own dimension. But in this case, the two languages agree: the heart is called mind and the mind is called heart, with (almost) no distinction.

The origin of the term *Kokoro* refers onomatopoetically to the heartbeat in the chest. It is therefore the centre of movement, the origin of natural life, the place where all breaths and essences come together to leave again.[2] By extending the meaning, it is everything that involves thought and spirit, and more specifically, intention in our actions. This is an important point, so important that in Asian medicine it is considered to be the Emperor, the highest figure in the inner empire that is our body. The role of the other organs is to execute, transport, transform, compare, discern and decide, but only the Emperor has an overall vision and remains the guarantor of order. What is this order? It's being in tune, in harmony with his regular beat, otherwise the whole thing will go haywire and risk coming to an abrupt halt. It is the celestial order that expresses itself through the Heart and sets the tempo, because the *Shén* we spoke of earlier, that spark of Pre-Heaven Essence (before birth), comes to find its home in the Heart.

The Heart governs and regulates the rhythm of life.[3] Beating long before birth, when Man is still only a foetus, and right up to the last breath, the Heart ensures the smooth running of the body-mind. It tells the individual how to proceed: neither too fast, nor too slow, and always with a happy intention. The Fire Element linked to the Heart shows that it is active, moving and, like Fire, can smoulder for a long time under the embers or become vast and even uncontrollable. The challenge for the mind is to understand what the Heart is saying, in order to balance emotions within the body-mind. While all the organs receive and process emotions, the Chinese classics of medicine state that only the Heart feels these emotions. This difference shows us once again that the Heart is the seat of the Spirit, a vast mind that encompasses both the intellectual and the emotional. Its main emotion is joy, but not just any joy: joy in and through action. This meaning is found in all the world's great religions and mysticisms. Feeling joy for nothing seems out of place. Hysterical joy suggests imbalance. Having no joy withers the individual and removes any desire to act.

In fact, when we are sad, we don't want to do anything but crawl back under the duvet and stop moving. On the other hand, if we exercise over a long period of time, the results we achieve bring us great joy. Climbing a mountain for days, studying an art for years, building a house with your own hands - all these things bring us the joy of having achieved something thanks to our intention turned into action. And that's the problem with our consumer society. It gives us the assumption that by giving in to our immediate desires, we can satisfy them and be happy. Yet the experience of consumerism consistently shows us that this is never the case. Every time desire is satisfied, the fire of the Heart is consumed. It is extinguished immediately, only to be vaguely rekindled, less and less strongly, at the next advertising solicitation. Without effort over time, this Fire has not built itself up: it's a straw fire that can't warm and nourish us from within. As a result, all we get is a pale copy of pleasure and joy, which vanishes in an hour or less. So, we have to start over and consume again, in a never-ending flight towards the illusion of happiness. That's the difference between being and having.

Every year I hear a student complain about the length and difficulty of studying Shiatsu. We have to recognize that Shiatsu, like meditation, like the martial arts, like the arts in general, is not a hamburger that we can eat in less than three minutes. It requires persistence, patience, courage, a strong and lasting intention, all qualities of the Heart. But what a joy it is to know that throughout our life we will be able to learn something without ever running the risk of becoming bored or repeating ourselves. That throughout our life we will seek to improve and deepen our gestures, our spirit, our awareness and our understanding of the world and the Universe. That throughout our life we're building ourselves up, strengthening ourselves, feeling life down to the very last detail. What a joy it is to follow our life's path with a clear mind, beat by beat.

So *Kokoro* gives us a sense of joy and action intertwined over time. But as the seat of the mind, it is the starting point of the intention that the practitioner gives to his gesture. In English, we have a number of expressions that explain what we should do with the Heart: "have your heart in the right place", "to have a heart of gold", "put your heart into doing something", "find it in your heart to do something", "follow your heart", "from the depths of your heart" and, perhaps the most beautiful, "to love with heart and soul". But it wouldn't be fair to forget the magnificent Japanese saying recalled by Shizuto Masunaga: "If the heart isn't in it, you can't see by looking, nor hear by listening." These expressions can all be applied to Shiatsu. They all speak of the quality of being that gives the correct intention. This correct intention is to be understood in the sense of the eightfold path in Buddhism, i.e., not to seek at all costs to do good according to precise rules, but to do what is right in each situation, for each person, at each moment. As the Heart is the seat of the Spirit that connects with Heaven, the intention is capable of adjusting and adapting to each moment. As the Heart has joy in action, it spontaneously directs the hands on what needs to be done to liberate and bring joy. As a practitioner, it's not uncommon to programme a plan of action and choose this or that meridian to help the receiver and then, along the way, realize that your hands are doing something completely different from what you had intended. Generally, at the end of the session, if we've let the hands follow their path away from our mind, the receiver expresses his pleasure by saying: "That was the best Shiatsu you've ever given me." This is always surprising to hear, but it shows just how important it is to let our hands act according to our Heart and not according to our mental patterns. As I have already said on many occasions and repeat here: "Hands without the Heart are dry."[4]

To sum up this dual function of the Heart-Mind, the great Zen master Shunryū Suzuki said:

> The mind that is always by your side is not just your mind, it is the universal mind, always the same, never different from another's mind. It is the Zen mind. It is a big, big mind. The mind is everything you see – this mind is in the same instant absolutely everything.[5]

During a trip to India where we were on a humanitarian mission for Shiatsu, Bernard Bouheret explained that the most important thing in a good treatment is to give the person joy. And putting his money where his mouth was, he gave me a wholehearted session. Before the hour was up, I was so full of joy that I was laughing to myself. The effect even lasted for several hours, and I laughed all the way to my bed; I fell asleep still laughing. That is the strength of a master: to be able to adapt to the recipient, to let your hands do the talking and to bring out the joy in the recipient. It takes time and hard work to reach this level. This joy is latent in all of us and is only waiting to emerge. Once it has been unearthed and brought to light, joy transforms and heals us. It's "the joy from the stars".

I shin den shin

The Japanese often use the expression *I shin den shin* to refer to the relationship between master and pupil, an expression whose meaning reflects a transmission that takes place directly "from heart to heart". At a certain stage, words are no longer useful. You have to know how to receive and therefore hear with your heart. Having this kind of relationship with a master is already a gift in itself. But in the Shiatsu giver-receiver relationship, exactly the same thing happens, including on an energetic level. There is no need to remind you that opening the Heart chakra in yoga and/or meditating on the Heart Sutra are fundamental steps in spiritual upliftment, but also in energy upliftment (they go hand in hand). As a result, Shiatsu – which involves both energy work and spiritual work – attaches immense importance to the Heart. Unfortunately, this dimension is rarely taught. Open any Shiatsu book (except for the book by the founder, Tenpeki Tamai, but it hasn't been translated) and you'll find everything about the technique, the smallest details, but almost nothing about the principles and even less about the language of the Heart, even though it represents the alpha and omega of our art. Take a complete beginner, have him touch a person towards whom he will send all his Heart. The receiver will be able to say that this is the most beautiful treatment he has ever received, whereas the beginner does not have the slightest hint of a technique.

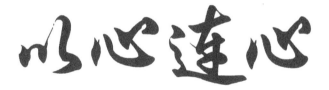

The *I shin den shin* relationship has a pitfall, a necessary pitfall for the pupil to mature. When a master takes a student close to him, the latter will quickly become astonished and then amazed by his master, his knowledge and everything he teaches him. If all goes well, he will spend his years of study with him in a kind of sweet euphoria, in which he will already be capable of doing a great deal. Once the student has his diploma, he will try to live the Shiatsu he has received. He will often not be as good as he was when he was just a student. He will also feel a loss of joy, enthusiasm or even empathy towards others. How can this happen? This is the moment of rupture, which is not easy for everyone. The teacher will be careful to cut the ties gently but firmly, so that the pupil can find out what he is really worth. And to do that, he will have to make the long journey to his own Heart, without being carried along by the inner strength and joy of his teacher. This is where the Way begins, a long journey full of doubts but oh so rewarding, where we learn that the most difficult trials are also the most formative and, in the end, the most rewarding.

Concerning I shin den shin, we often hear the following question in class: "How can we protect ourselves from bad energy?" For beginners, it's a good idea to explain a few techniques to protect oneself from the effects of perverse energy (Xié qì 邪气 in Chinese). But after a few years of practice, you must get rid of this vision and this approach. It doesn't help anything to hold on to the fear that a person's energy will rise into the practitioner's hands and then into his arms. On the contrary, you need to welcome this energy, which will then flow into the chest, pass through the Heart to be transformed and transmuted, and then flow back down the other arm towards the receiver. Why do you think we always work with two hands in Shiatsu? Because this creates a bridge, a bypass of Ki from one hand to the other and helps the person's energy to flow into their heart. You need to have a good heart, but above all you need the practitioner to have a strong centre. Strong from a cardiac point of view, strong emotionally (i.e., stable), strong from a compassionate point of view, non-judgemental and full of joy. This inner strength, which develops with personal work, with the journey over the years, enables the practitioner to receive all the energies there are, to transmute them and then to return them to their owner. This is where a heart-to-heart relationship is established. What's more, it's not unusual to see patients express gratitude, friendship and shared joy, even if this sometimes happens after tears.

How to develop the Heart?

Since no Shiatsu book seems to address the question in detail, let's ask how to develop the Heart? As with almost everything that affects the human being, we could mention, in no particular order, the love we receive from childhood, a balanced diet, a healthy lifestyle, a good night's sleep, parental education and the values passed on, life's encounters, experiences, learning, etc. In reality, human beings have only four primary needs: to have a roof over their heads to protect them from the weather and sleep peacefully; to have food and drink; to be at peace so that they can bring up their children and work or carry out their projects; to meet, talk, touch and interact with other people, because we are above all social animals. From then on, everything else – all the objects, pleasures and services to which we have access – should be seen as bonuses that enrich our enjoyment of life. But the consumer society has changed our perception of simplicity so that buying is the only solution to our happiness. Our hearts are therefore weakened by a fire without strength or flavour. Become aware of your primary needs and rejoice in having so much more. This change of perspective will once again open the way to satisfaction and joy.

Fortunately, there are many other aspects that strengthen the Heart. Contemplating nature is a primary and indispensable source of joy for filling and strengthening the Heart. We know, for example, that walking in the forest (*Shinrin yoku*, 森林浴: literally, forest bath) has become a discipline in itself in Japan. Not only do trees provide us with oxygen, but the half-light, the calm and the colour green all have a positive impact on the body and the spirit. Contemplation is a simple form of meditation that anyone can do. Who hasn't seen a breathtaking landscape, stopped talking, moving or driving to contemplate an ocean, mountains, a valley, a desert, a steppe or a field of flowers? According to the master Eckhart Tolle,[6] these are moments when the present is absolute, like a mini-*satori* that no thought disturbs. Meditation is another way of strengthening the Heart. By calming the maelstrom of our emotions and thoughts, the Spirit becomes clearer and can gently proceed to a clearer sense of the body and its capacities. As it passes through the Heart, it will feel a presence, a warmth and a strength that the individual did not know he or she had. The more a person meditates, the less agitation disturbs his inner lake and the more he will discern the important from the trivial. Then the Heart becomes as stable as an anchor, as strong as a mountain. There's no need to meditate for hours on end, but 15 to 30 minutes a day really makes a difference.

The gesture, the help, the gift, everything that comes spontaneously from within us is a real stimulant for the strength of the Heart. Nothing is worse than always calculating the benefits of our actions. To act freely and gratuitously without expecting anything is deeply soothing and satisfying. There's no need to be a great master here either. Every parent knows that children do this with grace when they offer a kiss, a drawing or a flower, and declare without batting an eyelid that Mum is the most beautiful person in the world. We are constantly interrelated with other human beings, and this dimension is highly nourishing when it is disinterested. We have to believe that the "social animal" side is only fully satisfied when it helps its neighbour.

Let's also consider the dimension of the Spirit in the Heart. Nourishing the Spirit should never be underestimated. There are many nourishments that the Spirit appreciates, starting with quiet reflection; quality reading where you can feel the author's benevolent intention through the words; taking the time to speak and act; learning by example and not by coercion; intelligent discussion with people who are advanced on a Way; prayer, whatever its form, belief or origin, as long as it promotes peace with oneself and with others; spending time with our loved ones; cultivating joy and all the emotions that feel good and do us good; the fundamental arts such as music, song and dance. These are – to contradict André Gide's key work[7] – our heavenly foods.

As Shiatsu practitioners know well, touch is an incredible way of soothing and strengthening the heart. But beyond the arts of touch, it's worth noting that a simple hug can go a long way towards soothing those who are suffering and strengthening the bonds of everyday life. On average, a hug lasts three to five seconds between members of the same family. A scientific study has shown that when this is increased to 20 seconds or more, hearts and breathing become harmonized and the entire sympathetic nervous system relaxes, while oxytocin levels rise.[8] Other, more disturbing studies[9] have shown that children who were not touched but fed by robots died quickly. Their hearts stopped, as if drained by a lack of presence and love.

Finally, let's not forget to mention empathy and compassion, which powerfully strengthen the Heart. We can think of religions, at least in their original form, because there is no human being who lives separately or above others. We are all interconnected through energy, Spirit, body and Heart. Being available for those who are suffering, helping the weak, the sick, the elderly and children, not making the neediest pay, all this gives the Heart the opportunity to express the nature of Heaven which, in return, will reinforce the power of the joy that dwells within us, in a virtuous circle that never stops. Thanks to Heaven, not only is the receiver strengthened, but the giver too, in a kind of cosmic game where everyone comes out a winner.

The beginner's heart

In all that has been said so far, one crucial concept is missing: *shoshin*. All the knowledge in the world in general and Oriental medicine in particular do not necessarily produce good results. Why is this? Because the mind is cluttered with knowledge that becomes certainty, and no longer listens to the heart. The Japanese, largely influenced by Zen, recommend applying *shoshin* to every course, every workshop, every practice. The beginner knows nothing yet, has no point of comparison and wishes with all his heart to learn again and again like a thirsty person.

Literally, *shoshin* is made up of two kanji: 初心. The first kanji 初 means "the first time, begin, start". It is itself made up of the radical for clothing 衤 and the kanji for knife or sword 刀. The second part is the heart kanji, which also designates the spirit in the symbolic sense, as "the Heart is the seat of the Spirit". Overall, it can therefore be translated as "the beginner's heart" or "the beginner's mind". Shunryū Suzuki Roshi writes that "in the beginner's mind there are many possibilities, in the expert's mind there are few. What is a beginner's mind? It's an open mind, an empty mind, a ready mind."[10]

The risk, then, is of getting stuck on your knowledge and not letting go. I'm quoting here from an extract on the same subject by Leo Tamaki Sensei,[11] founder of Kishinkai Aikidō.

> For an old hand, rediscovering *shoshin* is extremely difficult, but it's even more essential for progression. As the years go by, you naturally become familiar with the discipline you're studying. The environment of the dojo, the techniques, and the rituals of practice such as bowing become habits. And habit leads to automatisms. Automatisms that enable us to practise with greater ease and comfort.
>
> But that's also where progress often comes to an abrupt halt. And it can take months or even years to realize it. Some people become

complacent at this stage and may never even realize it. You'll find some amongst the elders in every dojo. Skilled and impressive at first sight, they are often role models with whom we identify. But following them can be dangerous because they are stuck at one stage and their understanding remains limited. The old-timer who questions himself and searches is a better role model, even if he may not be as flamboyant at first sight...

Easiness generally leads to pride. And habit constantly leads us to link what we see to what we already know. This is why the students of a master are often unable to follow him as he evolves. Stuck at a stage of his practice that they have mastered, they don't grasp the changes, looking at him today, but seeing what he did yesterday.

Some will never go beyond the stage of practice they have mastered and will continue indefinitely to refine techniques in intermediate work without moving on to the next stage.

Shoshin allows us to do each session as if for the first time, with a heart and mind (remember that both words are pronounced *shin* in Japanese) as fresh and new as the beginners. In this way, not only are you freed from all preconceptions, but *shoshin* also gives you a great deal of freedom to let your hands do as they please, without making any judgements about right or wrong. In this way, you are new every time and entirely available. Preciously cultivate *shoshin* within yourself, not only for Shiatsu but for every aspect of your life. The joy and inner freedom will be all the greater.

The heart of a mother

Shiatsu is a technique that has heart and comes from the heart. Never doubt this. This technique plunges to the source and returns to the source, passing from one person to another, from giver to receiver. So, it's not for nothing that Tokujiro Namikoshi said in 1968 what was to become his most famous quote: *Shiatsu no kokoro hahagokoro* ("The heart of Shiatsu is like the heart of a mother").

指圧の心は母ごころ圧
せば命の泉湧く
（ワツノハツノハ）

In a few words, this sentence sums up the very essence of Shiatsu: love (the heart of a mother), the technical principle (pressing) and its goal (bringing forth the springs of life). So, let's listen to this great master and look within ourselves for the heart that enables us to be a mother to humanity.

Summary

1. The Heart is the Emperor in Chinese medicine. It is at the centre of the emotions and the Spirit.
2. The relationship between a teacher and a student is heart to heart, not intellect to intellect.
3. It is vital to keep a new and open heart thanks to the beginner's mind.
4. Finally, developing the Heart in all its dimensions enables you to become a genuine and respectful practitioner.

27

Separation and Continuity

Tomorrow, at dawn, when the countryside brightens,
I will depart. You see, I know that you wait for me.

VICTOR HUGO (1802–1855)[1]

E very schoolchild in France knows these first two lines from *Tomorrow at Dawn*, one of the most famous poems by the great Victor Hugo. These two lines convey both the idea of departure and of reunion, and one might think that these words are contradictory. The answer lies in the rest of the poem, but from the point of view of Eastern thought, there is no contradiction here. As we have already seen, every thing, thought or movement has a complementary opposite, in other words a force that counterbalances and balances. And if there is a meeting, as we saw earlier, there is necessarily a separation. To put it simply, if there is a beginning, there is an end.

In martial arts, the Japanese use the concept of *Ki hazushi* (気外し) to refer to the moment when the two opponents separate at the end of the technique. In the Japanese language, it has the general meaning of disconnecting, disengaging, removing, detaching, all words that carry the idea of "undoing" or "breaking". It is a rupture that can be found at several points. First of all, it can be seen as a change of pace, a sudden acceleration that enables you to gain an advantage over the other fighter, or on the contrary, a sudden standstill that breaks the rhythm of the fight. It can also mean destructuring the opponent's body and energy. Finally, this expression is more simply used to describe the detachment and separation of the protagonists.

The art of separation

Let's quickly go back over the main principles that we have discussed, and which concern the relationship between the patient and the practitioner. *De-ai* (the encounter) consists of more subtle steps, including *Ki musubi* which creates a bond between people. Then the energy flows between bodies and minds with *Ki no nagare*, and finally both come to harmony with *Ki awase*. It is only because all these steps have been respected that a correct separation will be obtained where the actors of the meeting will both be satisfied, because mutually enriched by their respective presence and actions. But again, there is a whole art in the separation of bodies.

Take the example of the end of session. The hands placed on the body still take the time to give calm and presence. If at this moment we abruptly remove our hands, we get up and skip off to the toilet, it will be experienced as a brutal abandonment. The recipient will feel mistreated, forgotten or torn by this breakdown of energy. Let's start this step again, but this time in full consciousness. First of all, while leaving your hands where they are, start by coming to your senses, to identify yourself again as a person distinct from the other. Then bring your energy that wanders through the body of the receiver and again distinguish the border between your hands and the surface you touch. From there, lift very gently the heels of the hands and then the rest, in a movement towards the sky. Do not bring your hands back to you immediately but continue upwards in order to cross all the energetic layers and create a feeling of accompaniment. The movement of the hands is very similar to the first movement of the hands used in Tàijíquán. Therefore, put grace into this movement. The tranquillity and slowness favour the departure of the hands, a bit like a long goodbye when a friend puts his head through the window of the car, and then waves until you can no longer see him. Then, and only then, do a move just a little aside, thus regaining your distance to meditate, refocus or contemplate the relaxed face of the recipient. In fact, the most common reaction with this type of departure is:

"Oh, I thought you were still on my back/belly. I didn't feel you go." In fact, it's been a good five minutes since you stopped all movement. An angel passes by.

Now the question is: why do we have to take all these precautions? There are several answers to this.

- The simplest: because doing the gestures gently leaves precisely this impression in the body; leaving abruptly would waste all the work done before.
- The most energetic: because by doing so, we do not jostle all the energy layers that surround the body. Indian tradition talks about the seven layers of the aura.
- The most philosophical: because *Ki hazushi* is the opposite and complementary movement to *Ki awase*. *Awase* is a harmonious union movement and *hazushi* is its equally harmonious counterpart.

Never think that taking time to separate well is a waste of time. On the contrary, it is the best way to leave a person, while giving him the feeling that nothing stops. And that is exactly the objective.

Continuity in absence

Stopping the technique or the session does not mean that everything stops. Just like in sitting meditation, stillness does not mean the absence of movement. Don't judge a book by its cover. In Aikidō for example, we use the notion of *Kime* (決め), whose basic meaning is "locking". But it is interpreted as energy that continues its movement when one person has immobilized his partner. In Karate we speak of *Kime* as the spirit of decision. Nothing moves, but the energy, guided by the attention of the one who does the technique, continues and does its work. Here we find the relationship between *Qì* and *Shén* that we have already talked about. In Qìgōng, we voluntarily create pauses between sets of movements to feel the energy that continues its movement. At each pause we can identify the progression, strength and activity of the energy that grows in the body. We can find this feeling at the end of a good book or a movie as well. It is finished and yet, we have the impression of being carried on by the work, of living with it.

In Shiatsu, the same is true during breaks within the technique. This makes it possible to feel the energy acting without being distracted by the movement. This is particularly palpable after percussions. If these last at least five to ten minutes and they stop all at once, we can clearly feel a very tonic and almost "joyful" energy through all the muscles, meridians and even the bones. But we reach the top of our art when, at the end of the session, the person has the impression that you are still there. Better yet, the person will be able to tell you the next day all the effects they felt after your treatment. This can last up to three days. Post-treatment effects are divided into two stages. First, three days of the Yang phase which, as indicated by this type of energy, stirs and circulates until adopting a new body pattern. Then, three additional days of the Yin phase to integrate these changes, to the depths of our cells. Only after this six-day period can the person come back for another treatment, seven days after the previous treatment. This also explains why it is not recommended to do too many different treatments in the same week, for example a Shiatsu, an acupuncture session, and a visit to the osteopath. It is necessary to give the body time to integrate, to digest each session, and all of its mechanical, emotional or energetic information.

There is therefore a continuity of movement despite the end of the technique. We recognize great practitioners by the fact that we have the impression of always having their hands on our body hours after the end of the session. This presence is the continued work of energy which is only possible thanks to a very developed *zanshin* (thoughtless attention). Let us be clear: to achieve this result, the "technical technique" alone is not enough. The technique gives a framework, but it also locks the practitioner into this same framework. On the other hand, the intimate understanding of the principles developed throughout this book makes it possible to go beyond the technique, to free oneself from it. In other words, it is thanks to the principles that we move from the Shiatsu technique to the art of Shiatsu Dō. From now on it is no longer a question of pressing on a body, but of transmitting something larger that will make both the recipient and the practitioner grow.

Summary

1. As the start of a session and at the time of separation at the end, it is necessary to pay attention to the receiver.
2. The *Ki hazuchi* principle states that people should separate with awareness, tact and grace.
3. After the end is not the end. *Kime* is a notion where the actions and decisions of the practitioner continue his work in the body of the recipient.
4. The implementation of all the principles mentioned so far allows the continuity of Shiatsu after the Shiatsu.

Heaven

Philosophical Principles and Explanations

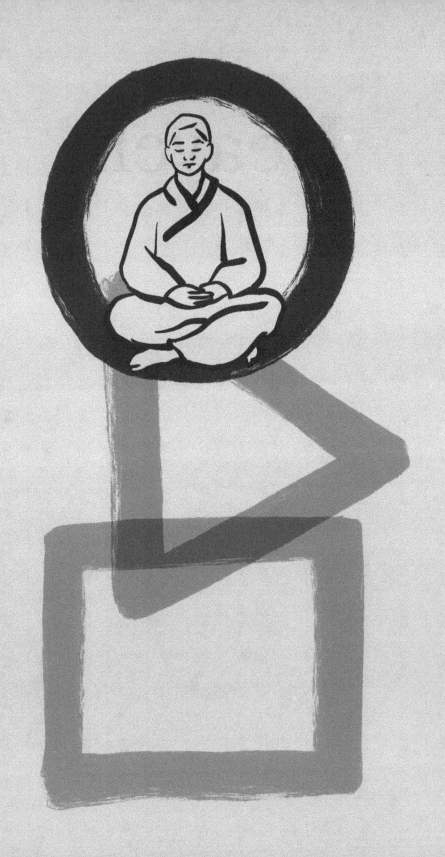

Explanation of the Philosophical Principles of the Shiatsu Way

I n this third part, we move away from the technique – as fine as it is – and the advanced concepts of the Japanese world to go towards the philosophy that underlies the art of Shiatsu Dō.

Dō, because it is indeed a Path and not a job, a Way of both natural health (from well-being to therapeutic), and also a Way of human development (for the practitioner as for the receiver). At the end of his course, no student can say that he has not changed one iota. Sometimes the transformation is going deep, so profound that it transforms the psyche, the body and the vision we can have of our world, our relationships, our lifestyles.

This change is driven by questions that affect us all from the depths of our humanity: Who am I? Why am I here and not elsewhere? What is the meaning of life? What is disease? How do the universe and the body work? What is the mind? Where do my thoughts come from? What are the interactions between environment and physiology, between physiology and psychology, between psychology and emotions? What is the point of spirituality? Is there a higher consciousness than my own consciousness? What is our place in the world? In the universe? And my place in society? Why does everything pass and change endlessly? Why do we have to die? What is reality? And so on.

Philosophy is the art of wisdom (*sophia*) through questioning and thought. Our ancestors from ancient Greece laid the groundwork for our Western way of thinking and were extraordinary pioneers. They asked themselves questions that no one before them had asked in such a systematic and pedagogic way. However, all human peoples did the same, to varying degrees, and with very different answers.

The fundamental questions of humanity are not foreign to Far Eastern thought, from India to Japan, Tibet and China. This thought is the very essence from which all the arts (martial, artistic or manual) draw their foundations and their wisdom. Of course, there are many books on these subjects, so many that we could spend a lifetime studying them without ever seeing the end. But in this section of this book, we will focus mainly on the philosophical principles found in the different currents of Shiatsu because, as Rabelais warned us: "Science without conscience will only ruin the soul."[1]

28

Macrocosm and Microcosm

The infinite universe
Through a small hole
Body of clay[1]

When talking about Oriental medicine, we cannot remove the individual physical body from the entirety of the universe. This is why the expression *ban butsu shō ō* (万物照応), which is translated as "everything is part of the whole", is of the utmost importance. To understand it, we need to widen our gaze to the widest dimension that our intelligence can embrace: the universe.

The universe is crisscrossed by electromagnetic waves and gravitational fields, as clearly demonstrated by Einstein and his followers. These waves carry information that will organize matter by making quarks and then atoms emerge. The latest theories about the universe explain that most of it is composed of dark matter that serves as a backdrop to the very structure of the universe. From this primordial soup[2] are created the first structures of matter, which at first hesitate between an organization as waves or atoms, exactly like photons of light, which are both waves and particles. Then these elementary particles, as for everything that surrounds us (water, fire, air, earth, plants, stones, metals, living beings), organize and densify, passing from the vaporous state of gas to that of dense matter.

For the ancient Chinese, the universe was One, a perfect unity but in which nothing moves. It is the *Tai kokyū* of the Japanese or the *Dào* of the Chinese. This unity breaks up to reveal two opposing and complementary forces (Yin and Yang, hot and cold, day and night, man and woman...) that move, repel and mate to create new elements. But every element of the great diversity of our world always contains the information of All. This is why everything is energy, because a pebble, a fish and a leaf are all made up of atoms and waves. Better still, they continue to receive waves from infinite space and to emit them because their atoms are also in constant motion, generating a signal. Matter is therefore both a receiver and a transmitter.

Man's place in this universe is the same – or almost the same – as that of the rest of nature. He is created as *Shén* or Spirit, which is the closest we know to the concept of the soul in the religions of the Book. The *Shén* is part of the Unity of the universe, in an area called the Prenatal Heaven or Pre-Heaven Essence, but has a consciousness of its own. As an integral part of Unity, it cannot experience diversity. To experience this, this *Shén* will transmigrate through the different stages of matter and finally incarnate in a body. This physical part of existence is called the Postnatal Heaven or the Post-Heaven Essence, which implies that before or after incarnation we are always and constantly connected to the Unity of Heaven, but in a different expression, a different form. This is how the heavenly *Shén* can experience matter, but also the multiplicity of things and therefore separation. It is also an often-cruel experience that we try to forget, especially by making love (fusion into the other) or by taking drugs (to forget one's physical dimension). Again, the *Shén*, incarnate as it is, will keep within it the notion of Unity of the universe, like everything that is composed of matter.

This very shortened and simplified explanation of Chinese thought on the notion of human being explains why our body is made up of atoms, receives and emits waves, and why logically it can only be made up of energy, like absolutely everything else around it. To remain consistent with its vision of the world (which is ultimately the same as our modern scientific vision, but 3000 to 5000 years ahead of it, depending on the source), Chinese medicine has chosen to intervene at the energy level, i.e., the vibratory level. Atomic medicine, like radiotherapy, deals with atoms. Allopathic and chemical medicine is concerned with molecules. Surgery, on the other hand, works at the level of matter, cutting to the quick. This shows that none of these medicines are perfect and that all are complementary to each other.

As proof, every change – natural or not – of chemistry of the body often modifies the psyche, that is, the Postnatal *Shén*, the one incarnated in the flesh. This is the reason why the side effects of certain medications can lead to depression for example. But according to the principle of back-and-forth and permanent movement of the universe (incarnation/movement/death/return to Oneness, then again incarnation, movement, and so on), if matter can influence the mind guided by the vibration of the original *Shén*, then the vibration of the original *Shén* can in turn modify matter, which in common language is called a miracle. In reality, this process is not miraculous, and it is not because we do not see something that it does not exist: think of the Emptiness of space, the air that we breathe, we can neither see nor grasp them, and yet... they exist.

If the vibrations of waves are used to organize matter, then this means that they carry structured and structuring information. In this way, by using the vibration of the mind, body and energy within us, Shiatsu practitioners (but also acupuncturists, magnetizers, etc.) can modify the vibrations of another person in order to bring them back into balance. This reasoning is implacable: as beings made of flesh and bone (and therefore of matter) we are both receivers and transmitters. The question that then arises is: what are we receiving? First of all, the vibration of our *Shén*, always connected to Heaven, whether before or after incarnation, and through this we receive the messages from the Unity, which can be interpreted as the rules of the game in which we evolve: the game of life, of course, as well as its creations, its forms and its transformations. Consequently, the imbalance of a human being, which is first vibratory, then energetic, psychic, psychological, physiological and finally mechanical, is above all a poor reception of the information from the Unity, and even more so a poor transcription and transmission to ourselves and to others. The causes of this poor reception/transmission (think of a crackling radio or TV set) are to be found in the loss of spiritual reference points that link us to the Unity, in the poor nutrition of the agro-industry that pollutes us, in the bad waves that parasitize us (Wi-Fi, satellite, mobile phones, power stations), in poor exchanges with others and with nature in general, in the fact of shutting ourselves away in our brain with the mind as our only reality without worrying about the body and, finally, in the fact of no longer receiving the reasons that pushed our *Shén* to incarnate. All these imbalances will disrupt the reception-emission process, and the material body will become profoundly disorganized. This is what we call illness.

Remembering that macrocosm and microcosm are intertwined is to say that everything that Heaven emits will change our balance... and it broadcasts continuously. There is an ancient Chinese saying that "from Heaven flows Virtue in a Yang movement", from top to bottom. For this broadcast to be beneficial to us (to stay healthy), the human being has the sacred duty to serve as a channel and interpreter between Heaven and Earth (or in other words between Prenatal and Postnatal Heaven), between the spiritual and the material. This was the role of priests in the first religions and of shamans still today. Without this, there will be no shortage of interference from reception and transmission, and the symptoms will arise, at first weakly, then more and more strongly, sometimes to the point of immobilizing or killing the defective organism because it is not respecting the rules of universal Unity. But while orders flow freely from Heaven to Earth, we must not forget that everything that happens on Earth also flows back up to Heaven in the form of information, in a Yin movement that takes the form of the "Ten Thousand Beings".[3] Mythological episodes such as the ten plagues of Egypt or the belief in the Apocalypse represent the punishment of men who have not respected Heaven.

In our bodily dimension, it's no different. The inexplicable illnesses which suddenly appear are generally slow, progressive evolutions which break through all the barriers of matter because the individual is no longer listening to his "mandate from Heaven", i.e., the reason why his *Shén* was incarnated. In the opposite direction, poor care of our bodily matter, from our tiny atoms to our major systems (endocrine, respiratory, digestive, etc.), lack of care for our psyche, our emotions, the absence of spirituality, will go right back up to the Heaven-linked *Shén* and make Man unhappy, depressed, anxious, even completely mad. That's why physical well-being and mental maintenance are the two basic keys to good health.

Macrocosm and microcosm are therefore one in the other, like Yin/Yang, inseparable, just as body and mind are. Until we have proof to the contrary, there isn't a metal plate separating our body from our head, is there? The study of Chinese medicine shows that the body itself is organized in this way. The proof is in reflexology. This technique considers that the ears (auriculotherapy), hands (palm reflexology) or feet (foot reflexology) each represent the whole body. The same principle applies to the nose, forehead, arms, legs and back – in short, every part of the body is a hologram of the whole. The undeniable success of these techniques, particularly in terms of well-being and health,[4] shows that the body can also be divided into microcosms that respond to the macrocosm of the body as a whole. Shiatsu books show that a hand is a microcosm, but so is a single finger, or even a single fingernail. There are microcosms such as the face (facial reflexology), the abdomen (used a lot in Shiatsu), the back, and so on. Physiological systems can also be read in this way, since everything is in everything. That's why observation and palpation are so important in Shiatsu, because they allow you – literally – to read a person beyond the words they speak.

At the source of energetics

For the Shiatsu practitioner, these notions of microcosm and macrocosm are crucial. They are found in all theoretical explanations such as Yin/Yang, Heaven/Earth/Man, the Four Seasons, the Five Movements, the Six Layers, etc. Indeed, they allow him to act on the whole of an individual simply by putting his hands on him and letting the vibratory energy pass massively to regulate the details of the body. Equally, he can also touch a microcosm to resonate the whole. This way of doing things is not the prerogative of Shiatsu; the healing touch can be found among Christians (it was also one of the qualities of ancient kings and especially of Christ himself, king of healers) and in many other traditions around the world. As the body is organized in microcosm-macrocosm, it will know how to take what it needs to get in tune (in harmony shall we say) with the information it receives from the microcosm (the practitioner) and the macrocosm (Heaven) above him.

In fact, this is the reason for using distal points in Oriental medicine. I experienced this following a traumatic accident involving my daughter. One of her playmates fell on her neck while she was swimming in a pool. The shock was such that she couldn't move at all, her neck hurting horribly. It was so sensitive that you couldn't even put your fingers on the skin of her neck. I wanted to relieve her, so I used the distal points reputed to treat the neck, and the corresponding foot reflexology zone. In just three days, she regained movement, and I was able to start treating the affected area more directly. But to use the distal points, I quickly realized that it wasn't enough just to press them – the human being isn't a computer with buttons to press – but to feel through them the connection with the suffering in the back of her neck. It's not very difficult to do: you just have to empty your mind and let the sensations come. Then, and only then, can the pressure of the fingers send information from a distance to relieve the pain.

The principle of interpenetration of the distant and the local, in other words of the microcosm within the macrocosm, is so powerful that the ancient Taoists classified different levels in the art of prac-tising Chinese manual medicine.[5] The lower one consists in treating the patient by touching him directly with the hands. The second one treats the patient without touching him, but by being next to him. The highest level is to treat the patient without touching him and at a distance. This last level uses the principle of resonance of energy that is everywhere, thanks to the connection between macrocosm (here the totality of our world) and microcosm (the specific individual). Needles and pharmacopoeia do not intervene until later, when a pathology is already well established in the patient. But the manual approach will always have precedence.[6]

Therefore, understanding the holographic principle that everything is in everything allows us to go to the very source of energy. If Shiatsu is not only based on the work of energy (there are also anatomical realignments, mobilizations and other aspects that we have already spoken of), it must be recognized that this consti-tutes a large part of its curriculum, especially since the writings of Shizuto Masunaga.[7] All that remains is to find the means to put all this into practice. There's no secret: you have to learn and work at it.

Summary

1. The macrocosm is made up of microcosms that react to it, and vice versa.
2. Waves are the medium of communication between macrocosm and microcosm.
3. The microcosm/macrocosm concept is tantamount to saying that "everything is in everything", the whole is in the detail, the drop of water contains the ocean.
4. Within the body, there are a host of microcosms that act on the whole. This is the principle behind the many systems used in reflexology.
5. Understanding and mastering this concept allows us to go to the source of how energy works.

29

The Environment and the Individual

Another closely related expression heard in Japanese schools of Shiatsu is *Shin do fu ni* (心土不二). Literally this means that "the Heart and the Earth are not two", but a better translation would be "a person and his environment are One". This notion is essential for understanding the interactions between the material world around us and how we function on all levels.

We are currently inundated with pathologies of all kinds, known modestly and fatalistically as "diseases of civilization". Among these, stress is of particular interest to us because, although it is not a disease in itself, it aggravates the majority of known diseases, if not all of them. To this we can add without hesitation all sorts of psychological disorders (neuroses and psychoses), physiological disorders (from rheumatoid arthritis to cancer) and even physical disorders (lower back pain, neck pain, wear and tear on joints and even bones). It's as if all these ailments just happened to fall into our laps, so we try to find remedies and carry on living as if nothing had happened, without changing anything.

As you will have understood, the body is both a microcosm of the universe and a macrocosm for our inner universes. As the Taoists so beautifully put it: "The body is a small universe and the universe is a large body".[1] We evolve in an environment that is at once the nature that surrounds us, the society in which we evolve, the culture that imposes its beliefs on us, and the family environment that greatly influences us. It is in the midst of all this that our physical body evolves and constantly responds to the information it receives.

We adapt to what we receive and, in return, send out just as much information. So, rather than believing in the inevitability of disease as a divine curse, it is more intelligent to rethink the interaction that exists between us and our environment. And yet, in our modern societies, what do we observe around us? Stress at work, an almost entirely destroyed and polluted natural environment, and a wide variety of beliefs that for centuries have led people to separate, hate and then kill each other. Fortunately, but very belatedly (too belatedly?), a wave of awareness has reached the thinkers about the importance of our environment. The loss of trees leads to the loss of arable land, which leads to famine and drought. Pollution from agro-industry and the modification of plant genes are leading to as yet unresearched changes in our own DNA and to a number of diseases including many forms of cancer.[2] Polluted water has depopulated our rivers and created acid rain, which not so long ago devastated the forests of Germany, Belgium and northern France. Our vegetables and fruits no longer grow freely, nourished only by the blessings of the Earth and the Sun, but forced into hydroponic greenhouses with only nutrients distilled in a water-like liquid, a kind of synthetic syrup full of artificial additives. It is obvious that our body reacts, and rather badly, to these disorders that parasitize our biology.

Unfortunately, the list of parasites that keep us off the path to good health is almost endless. The clothes we buy are full of insecticides, nanoparticles, aluminium and soon, internet-connected electronics. The food we buy is full of pesticides, additives, sweeteners, preservatives, and therefore endocrine disruptors, with the serious consequences we know about for our hormonal glands, such as the alarming drop in fertility in men and in women, as well as all the foetal malformations. Our homes are so well insulated that there's no draught to blow away dust mites, pet saliva, piles of dead skin, or aerate the chemicals in household products. No wonder children are increasingly allergic. The waves from our smartphones, DECT base stations, microwave ovens and other Wi-Fi hotspots (the one in our house and the 20 or so others in the neighbourhood) are so present that a federal and official US study in 2016 clearly indicated the risks of brain and heart damage.[3] The litany could go on and on. And people are surprised when they "fall" ill.

It's our natural environment that we've profoundly disturbed. These imbalances, the pollution we produce, are all unhealthy information that flood our Earth. As we are the mediators between Heaven and Earth, this information also pollutes us, and we are also the sufferers of this situation. Eastern medicine has been explaining this interrelation for millennia, but it's not the only one. Didn't the founding father of Western medicine, Hippocrates, to whom doctors take an oath, declare: "Let food be thy medicine, and let medicine be thy food"?

But how can we heal ourselves with such bad food? Faced with this breakdown in our environment, it is more than urgent to treat the world in which we live as well as our minds, since one cannot exist without the other. Of course, we can give up, but then diseases will only increase (you can bet on it with certainty) and the pharmaceutical industry has understood this. Or we can choose to take charge of our own health, as, fortunately, more and more people are doing.

Taking back control

Of course, taking back control of our environment means eating organic and local produce, reducing pollution as much as possible, and choosing merchants who are worthy of receiving our money. On an individual level - and of direct concern to Shiatsu practitioners - we also need to act for our health, particularly regarding our diet. Our bodies get their energy from three sources: air, food and drink, and energy.

- **Breathing** is the first and last activity of our life on earth. It is both a means of oxygenation and of expelling carbon dioxide from our bodies. It is also an excellent way of calming mental agitation. That's why everything from meditation to dance, yoga and the martial arts is all about breath (in every sense of the word). What all these arts have in common is that they put the body back at the centre of attention, without going through the mind. In this way, we are reminded that we are alive thanks to our entire physiology and not just our thoughts.

- Once this awareness has been established, **food** becomes the best way of balancing our bodies. Not only must it be as pure as possible (excluding pesticides is a minimum), but it must also be as balanced as possible. For millions of years, our bodies have adapted to the changing seasons. That's why it's so important to eat fruit and vegetables in season. What's more, in summer our bodies need vitamins because they move around a lot. In winter, on the other hand, we become more static; for its maintenance and endurance, the body needs mineral salts above all. As chance would have it, summer produces sun-drenched, above-ground fruit and vegetables, which enable vitamins to be synthesized; in winter, vegetables in the ground draw a maximum of mineral salts from the earth. After that, there are many different ways of eating, many different diets, and so on. But the most important thing is always to avoid food from the agro-industry, which is inevitably processed and manipulated and contains many chemical agents and additives. Listening closely to our bodies (and not to our immediate cravings) helps us to know what we need, especially when we no longer feel like eating and our spirits are high. It's about the need to purge and do a little rejuvenation, a process that has been ritualized in all the world's religions, no matter what type.
- Finally, the third necessity for regaining control of your health is to maintain and improve **the movement of energy**. As matter and energy are one and the same – or two sides of the same coin – moving your body enables you to activate your energy dynamically. The body needs both physical exercises to toughen up, resist and sweat[4] (through what we commonly call sport) and flexibility exercises (to keep the joints in good condition and avoid the joint injuries so common with age). As the anatomists say, "the only way to prevent wear and tear on the body is to use it". Through physical activity, we consume matter (gas, solid and liquid food) and transform it into energy that enables mobility and effort.

Healing the Shén

To paraphrase Mahatma Gandhi, it is a fundamental truth that every soul who raises themselves, raises the world.

The three aspects listed above are the basis for taking back control of what we ingest, i.e., the information provided by the Earth. But all too often, many people stop at this observation. Admittedly, they feel better for a while. And yet, despite having everything they need to be happy, they come to a Shiatsu session with their spirits in the dumps. Clinical experience shows – and this is the great novelty of the last ten years – that people don't come just to be free of pain, but to find an answer to their distress, to their illness.

The question of meaning is now at the heart of the disease's process. If the practitioner can explain that food is not only earthly but also celestial, then a new door is opened in the spirit's understanding. Because that's what it's all about: spirituality. Health depends not only on the earthly environment but also on the heavenly one.

- The first heavenly necessity – which we urgently need today – is the cleansing of the mind. We are constantly evolving in a world of thoughts, reflections, analyses, readings, conjunctures, ponderings and viewings, all of which are activities of the brain. And to rest, many people, starting with the youngest, take refuge in virtual worlds (imaginary, chemical, computerized or televized). But the brain and its activity (the mind) are not the only dimensions we possess. The brain is the zone of our structured thoughts, our conscious mind, our on-board computer that manages the details of our organism. Meditation allows us to see that it is just that: a super-computer, a tool that may be ultra-sophisticated, but it's just a tool. And we have let the tool become the master by abandoning the command post. In meditation classes, I often tell students that they're like empty houses, with only the bluish screen of a computer that's gone mad because it's running on a loop with no one to direct it. Meditation allows us to calm the endlessly spinning programmes and to rediscover the different parts of ourselves: the body, the mind, the heart and the spirit. Just as everything we are influences our bodies, our thoughts also have this capacity, for good or ill. Everyone has already seen the catastrophic effect of negative thoughts on health, otherwise psychotherapy and psychoanalysis would not have been invented.

- The second celestial necessity is to pay close attention to our emotions. Emotions are intense movements of energy between our mind and our body, in other words between our individual Heaven and our personal Earth. We can think of them again as information waves, but at a high frequency. There's no need to describe what triggers love, pain, joy or anger. What's more, we still don't really know why we fall in love suddenly. The Chinese speak of a message from Heaven. As Shiatsu practitioners, it's interesting to note that the five basic emotions linked to the Five Movements are joy, sadness, anger, introspection/reflection and fear. Our personal work consists of balancing them without giving preference to one or the other. Thanks to this, the inner disturbances are less significant when they are transmitted, so the body's reactions are not as strong when they are received. This reduces the risk of developing physiological or mechanical problems resulting from strong emotions. Emotional transmitters can also be people in our private or professional environment. Calming our emotions also helps us to avoid over-investing in other people's emotional outbursts. A colleague who loses his temper is not necessarily angry with us; he is probably frustrated or unhappy elsewhere.[5] We don't need to take it personally and carry their problem. Let's not forget that an emotion is a wave of energy that vibrates strongly, as much as words and gestures, if not more. In this way, we can let emotions slide over us and not make them our own, and not carry the burden of others, which is crucial in the role of the Shiatsu therapist. Your mental, emotional and energetic health is at stake.

- The last heavenly environment we need to get back in hand to improve our health is our beliefs, most of which are prejudices. Racist, religious, sexual preference, gender, cultural, caste or group, scientific, mythological – the list of prejudices goes on. One example: for a long time it was believed that women could not do the same jobs as men. Today they occupy the whole range of existing professional positions, even the most arduous (coal miners) or the most destructive (soldiers), without this being a problem for them. These prejudices are also present in our individuality: believing ourselves to be incapable, bad lovers, indestructible, superior to others, less than nothing, stupid, etc. These beliefs are largely harmful to our psychology because, like all beliefs, they shape us and become an integral part of our personality. In meditation, teachers ask: "Does this belief make you happy? No?! So, change it." The role of the Shiatsu practitioner is exactly the same. He must offer the receiver the opportunity to change his beliefs so that he is no longer stuck in a sclerosing system that stagnates his psychic energy and traps him in physical discomfort. To achieve such a result, the practitioner himself must continually cleanse himself of his beliefs to be open to all the messages from Heaven, the essence of which can be summed up as follows: Love.

Cleaning up society

Each individual therefore vibrates in unison with terrestrial and celestial information. But the human group, society as a whole, is also an environment to be reckoned with. This is why Kawada Sensei spoke in his classes of "people's karma". A society as a whole vibrates and gives off a certain energy. And each individual is, once again, both the receiver and the sender of this society, in this microcosm-macrocosm relationship that we continually find. Of course, a society at war does not emit the same vibration as a society at peace, and its individuals are therefore not in the same state of physical and psychological health. Every society is also made up of beliefs and therefore prejudices. Some of its beliefs lead into hellish spirals of unhappiness and even self-destruction;[6] current events provide us with constant sad examples of this. On the other hand, some societies aim for well-being, such as the Scandinavian countries and Bhutan, which, in 1972, was the first country to calculate its wealth in terms of Gross National Happiness (GNH).

It doesn't take much imagination to see the implications of such decisions on the vibration of individuals, and therefore on their health. Individuals are like leaves on a tree. They are all independent and each vibrates in its own way; but at the same time, they are all connected to a single branch (society) that vibrates in unison, which in turn is connected to the common trunk that is humanity. Once more, we see the relationship between microcosm and macrocosm. In terms of our inner environment, it's exactly the same situation. The acupuncture points (or *tsubos*) vibrate independently, but all are linked to a meridian which vibrates in unison with all its points, and all the meridians are linked to the common trunk that is the individual. This is why the vibration found in each *tsubo*, or in a person as a whole, amounts to one and the same piece of information: the state of energy and therefore the state of health. To understand this is to understand the importance of the relationship between the individual and his or her environment, the grail being to become one, to rediscover the unity between our nature and Nature.

It is interesting to note in passing that Taoist philosophy, itself derived from shamanism and animism, is an ecosystem of the inner and outer environment. It is a constant reminder of the relationship between the being and its environment, nature and the human being who inhabits it, in a closed cycle, as we will see in Chapter 31 on the circle and the spiral.

Anyway, if each leaf on the tree can clean itself, improve itself and purify itself, then the whole tree that bears them will shine again. If each individual takes charge of his or her life and stops relying on solutions outside the body-mind, society as a whole will improve and become a haven of peace and light for all. In other words, every microcosm can change the macrocosm of society. But it is also possible to change the macrocosm. First, by choosing political representatives who propose to look after the environment and citizens, reduce inequalities, redistribute wealth, protect the weakest – in short, become virtuous, as Confucius advocated to the princes of predynastic China.

In 2015, during a visit to Brussels, Tshering Tobgay, the Prime Minister of Bhutan, told the leaders of the European Union:

Why govern if not to make people happy?[7]

Summary

1. The environment, nature, has a direct influence on human beings.
2. Individuals must take charge of their health by taking care of their breathing, diet and physical activity.
3. The mind needs to be calmed so that the Spirit (*Shén*) regains its radiance and doesn't sink into a psycho-emotional turmoil.
4. Every individual who improves himself changes the society around him. But it is also possible to modify society as a whole in order to heal its individuals. To paraphrase Gandhi, Every soul that raises itself, raises the world.

30

Everything Is Movement

Complementing the previous notions, the third philosophical statement is *Banbutsu ryūten* (万物流転). This famous expression states that "everything is movement".[1] It is quite easy to understand this statement nowadays, with ecological awareness and education about ecosystems. The elements of an ecosystem are both interconnected and in motion. Heraclitus of Ephesus (of the pre-Socratic school, 544 to 480 BCE) already expressed it in the formula *Panta rhei* (Πάντα ῥεῖ): "all things flow" or "everything moves according to a certain rhythm". And we cannot forget to quote this sentence by the same author: "You never bathe in the same river twice."

Let's take nature as an example. For a long time, many insects were considered pests. Within a generation, their eradication with DDT led to the disappearance of many of the birds that lulled the ears of our parents, such as the nightingale, the chaffinch and even the skylark. In other natural environments, the disappearance of super-predators such as the wolf, the tiger and the shark leaves the way clear for their prey to multiply unregulated and invade human cultures or their environment. This is the case in France, where despite the increase of hunting rights, wild boar and deer have never been so numerous, eating crops to the great displeasure of farmers.[2] It is the principle of interrelation – and therefore of balance – that is undermined each time, causing new evils that are getting worse and worse. This brings to mind a quotation from Laozi, the father of Taoism:[3]

Happiness is based on unhappiness,
Unhappiness broods beneath happiness.
Who knows their respective peaks?

The principle of movement is inherent to life in matter. Everything has a material beginning and end, even mountains. We are all born and we all die or, as the Dalai Lama says, "we all have the same origin and we all end in the same way".[4] In between, we move left and right, here and there, thanks to our locomotor system. The water that falls from the sky, then from the mountains, runs down to the sea before evaporating and leaving again in the form of clouds. Our thoughts come and go by the thousands in a single day (an average of 60,000 a day), as do our emotions. Atoms move everywhere, in all directions, within us and all around us. Everything is in motion. If we don't respect this principle, we're heading straight for a dead end, from which will arise a malaise that will quickly turn into an illness. Let's take an example that we've all seen or experienced at least once: a love relationship. In a love relationship, as the years go by, many people try to freeze the relationship as it was at the beginning, to find and keep the spark that made their heart leap. It's obviously an illusion to believe that this is even possible for a moment. It's the same with a break-up. Many people refuse to accept the break-up and shut themselves away in denial, loneliness and sadness. In both cases, suffering is the result.

It is sometimes possible to block the principle of flow, but this is always to the detriment of health. To entrench yourself in this situation is to commit yourself to suffering and exhaustion. This is what happens to the lovers in the previous example. Now imagine that we are big and strong enough to block the flow of water like a dam. What is going to happen? The water will go stale, then rot and become mud, making way for all sorts of unpleasant plants and smells, becoming the swamps that our ancestors rightly shunned as unsanitary and sources of disease. A person who tries (consciously or unconsciously) to freeze a situation, an emotion or a will provokes exactly the same results in his personal ecosystem.

So, what is the solution? Buddhism offers a very interesting answer: letting go. This posture means that under no circumstances should you block anything. Time, for example. We all grow old. Fighting against time with anti-wrinkle cream or cosmetic surgery changes nothing. On the contrary, it will make us suffer a little more each day as we look in the mirror. On the other hand, accepting time and our mortality means that we don't need to fight against the movement of life, because that's the golden rule of the matter that makes us up; the better to decompose. Better still, swimming with the current is the art of saving energy. This is the whole point of energetic exercises, the cleansing we have mentioned and the management of body and mind. In this respect, it is interesting to read the first lines of the classic of Chinese medicine, the *Huángdi Neijīng*, or *The Yellow Emperor's Internal Classic*. It states:

> *I've heard it said that men of old*
> *Lived to be a hundred,*
> *Always active, unaware of senescence.*
> *But today's men*
> *Are old men at fifty.*
> *Are today's generations different*
> *From the old ones?*
> *Or has the human race lost something?*

Many people today complain that things were better before. It's amusing to read that 2000 years ago people didn't think any differently. Emperor Huang Di complained that no one knew how to stay healthy and grow old. To which the Taoist master Qi Bai, who was also his minister and personal physician, replied:[5]

> *The men of old*
> *Were wise men who obeyed the Tao,*
> *The universal law of Yin-Yang,*
> *The only possible rule of life.*
> *[...] They understood the relationship between body and mind.*
> *Between body and spirit.*

Later in the book, *Qi Bai* concludes that the solution lies in the use of needles and moxas (terms used in Chinese medicine) and in respect for nature. Now, I'm deliberately repeating myself; the primary rule of nature is movement. But the poet Li Bo[6] expressed it even better when he compared the universe to:

> *An inn, a place of incessant comings and goings,*
> *where people come and go without interruption.*[7]

So, as the Buddha teaches, we have to accept. Accept that we are all subject to the passage of time and to ageing, to the illness that will come our way one day or another, to the death that will take us. There's the now famous anecdote of a psychiatrist who shows a glass containing a little water to her audience at a major conference. Everyone expects the classic question of whether the glass is half full or half empty. But she surprises her audience by asking: "How much does this glass weigh?" And then everyone comes up with their own estimate. But she replies that it doesn't matter. The only risk is keeping it in your hand for too long. After three minutes, her fingers will feel stiff. After ten minutes, her shoulder and arm will start to stiffen. After several hours, she'll trigger all sorts of tension traumas from her fingers to the base of her skull and probably beyond. Within a day, her mind will be screaming and her whole body will be shaking. The only right answer is to drink the contents of the glass, enjoy it and be happy with it, then quickly put the glass back down because life must go on. Otherwise, it's just suffering. That is letting go. Putting down your baggage, your desire, your trauma, your worry, your unspoken words, so that you can get on with life and bathe in it with joy.

Movement in the Five Phases

Without movement, there is no life. From man to woman, from sperm to egg, from water to cells, from Heaven to Earth, from winter to spring, from Yang to Yin, from light to shadow, all speak of movement. The Taoist philosophy that underlines Oriental medicine is made up of many theories, but of all of them, that of the Five Elements is undoubtedly the most telling. In fact, specialists don't like to talk about the Five Elements, because it gives the false idea that they are fixed in matter. Instead, we speak of the Five Movements or the Five Phases of transformation. Wood expands in all directions, Fire rises towards Heaven, Metal tightens and condenses inwards, Water insinuates itself and descends to the depths, and Earth remains at the centre and brings stability to the other movements. Note that the Earth is not immobile because it is at the centre. Remaining centred represents an effort and a constant movement from oneself towards oneself.

These Five Movements are represented in the form of a cross (representing the material world horizontally and the spiritual world vertically) or in the form of a circle, with which all Shiatsu students are familiar. This pattern is known as the "generation" or *Shēng* 生 cycle. Wood nourishes Fire; Fire becomes ashes, which nourish Earth; Earth condenses, giving rise to ores, and therefore to Metal; Metal can melt and become liquid, but it also concentrates the morning dew, so it engenders Water; and Water makes vegetation grow, i.e., Wood. It is this movement of generation from one Element to another that makes life possible. But to maintain the balance of the whole, a second cycle is superimposed to control the Elements, also called the *Ke* 克 cycle. The term "control" is not entirely correct, because while the Elements do indeed control each other, they also help each other when there is a deficiency. Wood controls Earth to prevent it from eroding (the roots hold back the soil); Earth holds back Water (to prevent flooding); Water calms the burning of Fire (and keeps it within its limits); Fire melts Metal (to prevent it from cutting everything); Metal cuts Wood (so that vegetation doesn't invade everything and leave no room for man to grow crops). These relationships form a pentagram at the centre of the circle of generation. Balance therefore involves a simultaneous double movement: external and visible, with the wheel generating and creating movement (this is the Yang principle); internal and invisible, with the spokes reinforcing and maintaining the relationships, cohesion and potentiality of movement (the Yin principle). These two cycles are inseparable and complementary.

The five antique Shu

Thanks to this theoretical structure, all practitioners of Oriental medicine (acupuncturists, doctors, herbalists, massage therapists, Qìgōng masters) can understand the root of imbalances in an individual's health and develop a treatment strategy. For example, if Fire is absent, the person will be sluggish, lacking in the desire to move or take action, and be quite depressed. Stimulating the generating and supporting relationships, i.e., stimulating Wood and Water, can nourish Fire and restore the person's desire to live. This principle of the circulation of energy between the movements of nature is also present within the organs, the channels and even the points known as the five antique *Shu* points.[8] The macrocosm–microcosome principle is still at work. These antique *Shu* points are decisive in the first therapeutic level of Shiatsu, and I refer the reader to Michel Odoul's excellent explanation on this subject.[9] Each of these five points represents an Element and, for each channel, two of them constitute the toning point and the annual dispersion point of the energy of the said channel. Mastering these ancient *Shu* points is complex, and there are several ways of using them. The Japanese, who are the great champions of the Five Movements theory, link them to Wood, Metal, Water, etc. However, the Chinese, who developed this system, speak of the principle of flow. At the end of a channel, the first point is the well point (*Jǐng*, emerging from the depths of energy); the second represents the spring (*Yíng*, the spring that gushes forth); the third is the stream (*Shū*, the energy is stronger); the fourth the river (*Jīng*, the energy is greater); and the fifth the sea (*Hé*, the energy is deep, it sinks into the meridian). This image of water rising up, flowing down to the sea and gaining in intensity (quantity of energy) and depth (quality of energy) makes it clear that energy must circulate, it must move, to provide the body with the quantity and quality essential for life in good health. Regarding pathology, the classics of Chinese medicine teach that energy progresses in the body from the starting point *Jǐng*, gradually sinks in until it reaches the point *Hé*. It is considered easier to stop a pathology when it is still weak at the first points than at the end of the flow where it is difficult to stop once it has reached the depths. As soon as the pathology passes the Sea point (located on the elbow or knee), it attacks the organ linked to the channel. Here again, we can clearly see the idea of movement, both in health and in the worsening of the disease, from its first symptoms to its outbreak.

And this image of the movement of water doesn't stop there. In fact, the antique *Shu* organize the Elements in a different order depending on whether it is a Yang or a Yin channel.

- **Yang channel**: Metal → Water → Wood → Fire → Earth
- **Yin channel**: Wood → Fire → Earth → Metal → Water

However, this order poses a problem. Yang is traditionally associated with heat, the Sun and Fire, and Yin with coolness, the Moon and Water. So why start with Metal for the Yang meridian and Wood for the Yin meridian? In his excellent course on Oriental medicine, Jean-Marc Weill[10] explains that the answer lies in the movement of energy. The image he uses is that of a great river and its tributary, such as the Saint Lawrence and the Saguenay in Canada. The difference in flow and water quality means that the glacier-blue water of the Saguenay does not mix with the muddy water of the St Lawrence at the point where the two rivers meet. For another ten kilometres, the inertia of the rivers is such that the two waters flow together without mixing. Then the waters finally merge. The same is true of energy, which is nothing but movement. The Yang channel starts with a Metal point, which is like the meeting point of the two rivers, Yin and Yang. Then, when the energies merge, at the second antique *Shu* point, it feeds on the Element of the opposite channel, i.e., in the Yin channel, the Fire point. In this way, Metal finds the Fire it needs for its Yang quality. And the reverse also works, since the starting point of the Yin channel is Wood, which goes to the second point of the Yang channel to find the Water element, the quality necessary for the expression of Yin.

This is why the five antique *Shu* points were one of the first treatment systems in Chinese medicine, offering direct, practical access to the Five Movements and the ability to balance Yin/Yang energy. They also demonstrate that in the macrocosm of nature, as in the microcosome of a channel, everything is movement, and that movement is the basis of all life. Moreover, every theory of Chinese thought (Yin/Yang, Earth/Man/Sky, the Five Phases, the Six Layers, the Eight Directions, etc.) is based on the principle of movement, relationships and exchanges. Consequently – and quite logically – the Chinese vision of health could only be a relational and dynamic medicine, the opposite of modern, scientific medicine, which separates and analyses on the slides of a microscope. If relationships break down, imbalances appear. If this movement is interrupted, illness will arise.

276 THE SPIRIT OF SHIATSU

Summary

1. In the universe, everything is motion; therefore, life is motion, from beginning to end.
2. It is as pointless as it is impossible to stop movement; when this happens, illness gradually sets in.
3. *Ki* is like water; it must always be in motion.
4. The theory of the Five Movements is the best illustration of this.
5. The points of the five antique *Shu* are the concrete application of the previous theory; they act directly on the movement of *Ki*.

31

The Circle and the Spiral

The infinite circle is a classic of Japanese Zen painting.[1] A perfect line, an object of inspiration and meditation, it is also an extremely difficult exercise for the painter or calligrapher. Drawing a circle freehand is not at all easy with a simple pen. With a brush it is even more difficult, and you need total commitment of body, breath and mind to hope to succeed.

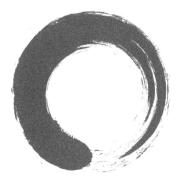

This circle is generally not closed so that we can see the brushstroke, its evolution from beginning to end, and, through this, the strength and presence of the artist. What the line suggests to the observer is the force of movement in the circle. Once again, everything is in the whole, the environment and the individual are one and all is movement. This movement, like the drawing of the circle, shows that all the facets of nature form a cycle. You can just think about the cycle of days, seasons and years, the Moon around the Earth, the Earth around the Sun. All these cycles follow one another in a long ascending then descending movement, called "life".

For Shiatsu practitioners, cycles are at the heart of their under-standing and practice. There are many of them: the cycles of the nine major physiological systems (bone, circulatory, digestive, respiratory, uro-genital, nervous, musculo-tendinous, lymphatic, endocrine), cer-tain more specific cycles (cells, embryogenesis, body fluids, blood), but even more so the cycles of energy. As every Shiatsu student in the world quickly learns, energy peaks and travels through a channel in two hours, one hour rising and one hour falling, before moving on to the next channel. This does not mean that the other channels are not irrigated, but simply that each meridian has a two-hour peak of activity. Energy starts in the chest, moves up to the hands, then from the hands to the head, from the head to the feet, and from the feet back to the chest. After four channels, energy has circled the whole body in eight hours. It then moves on to the next four channels in the order of the Chinese body clock. This complete circuit of the body also forms two cycles of energy that irrigate the body every four hours via a pair of channels. These are known as the Six Levels, which represent different energy potentials. These levels are called *Taiyīn* (great Yin) and *Yángmíng* (bright Yang), *Shaoyīn* (little Yin) and *Taiyáng* (great Yang), *Shaoyáng* (little Yang) and *Juéyīn* (finishing Yin). In other words, a complete circuit of the body allows two of these qualities of energy to develop through specific channels.

After three complete circuits of the body, 3 x 8 hours, a 24-hour day is completed, an entire circadian cycle.[2] As there are 12 channels and each has a two-hour peak of energy activity, there are 12 x 2 hours, again 24 hours. We can also calculate in the following way: 6 qualities of *Ki* x 4 hours = 24 hours. It all adds up. Then we start again with a complete round the next day from 3 a.m.

However, if we try to link the 24 hours – i.e., the 12 channels x 2 hours – to the natural forces of the Five Elements, we seem to find ourselves at a dead end, since 5 Elements x 2 hours only comes to 10, not 12 channels. The Oriental mind is not bothered by the problem of Cartesian thinking and always finds a solution for what is – appar-ently – illogical. Within the Five Movements, Fire has a special place and does not have just two channels, but four, divided into Emperor Fire (H-SI) and Minister Fire (PC-TB). The importance given to Fire (which animates, warms, and circulates thoughts and emotions) indicates that it is the key element in the human being. With a body temperature of 37°C on average, incessant thoughts, good locomotor mobility and a multitude of emotions, human beings need a lot of Fire to perform on a daily basis. Thanks to this little explanation of human nature, the cycle does indeed include five movements and 12 channels, without this being a problem, quite the contrary. So, we have come a full circle.

The cycle of the seasons is not a problem for a Western mind. Each season has three months, so 4 x 3 months make 12 months, or a full year, and that's all there is to it. This is to forget a little too quickly that it is the Chinese spirit that presides here. Each season is linked to one of the five movements of nature. Spring is linked to Wood, Summer to Fire, Autumn to Metal and Winter to Water. This cycle of seasons does pose a problem. Once again, how can we link four seasons with five movements? For the Chinese mind, we mustn't forget that nature is in constant motion, so this is not a problem of logic but of an intimate understanding of nature. The Earth element represents calm, the centre, immobility, the moment of reflection and introspection. Consequently, the wise man who follows the rhythm of nature knows that going from one season to the next requires a break, due to the risk of exhaustion (which is common in our society, resulting in chronic fatigue and complete exhaustion). As a result, the Chinese cycle of seasons cleverly proposes a return to the Earth at each inter-season (the fifth season), to regain strength and take stock of what has been achieved and what remains to be done before embarking on a new active phase. There's a saying that sums up this period very well: "sorting the wheat from the chaff" – taking the time to sort out the good from the bad experiences before embarking on a new cycle, a new season. So, for nine days at the end of one season and nine days at the start of the next (an inter-season of 18 days), the Earth makes its influence felt. In this cycle, there are therefore four seasons of 73 days (= 292) and four inter-seasons of 18 days (= 72), making a total of 364 days. The remaining day is of no interest to the Chinese because their calendar is lunisolar and works differently from ours. On the other hand, these inter-seasons are of particular interest to Shiatsu practitioners, as they always represent a delicate moment for closing the energy of the ending season and preparing the body for the energy of the following season, not to mention refocusing and strengthening the individual via the Earth (in other words the Stomach and Spleen).

Far from being an intellectual pastime, the understanding of these cycles allows the practical application of strategic choices to rebalance an individual, to put him back in the cycle of nature, nature of which his body and mind are part. This is why the notion of cycle is so important. But this is only the first step towards a more advanced understanding. That is what the cycle of the Essence teaches us.

Ki or *Qì* (energy) flows through the 12 main channels, and this notion is now widely popularized by health, wellness or women's magazines. On the other hand, few people know that at the root of *Qì* is *Jīng* or Essence, which is a more condensed form of energy. To understand the difference between *Jīng* and *Qì*, we can use the image of cooking gas. This gas can be liquid (compressed in a cylinder) and therefore have a high density, but to be ignited it must become lighter, more vaporous, through a regulator and, therefore, be able to circulate faster. From the decompression of *Jīng* (the liquid gas of our allegory) via *Huǒ ming mén* (火命门), the Fire of the Gate of Life[3] (the regulator), *Qì* is created. Be careful, this does not mean that *Jīng* precedes *Qì*; the two are connected and *Qì* is also present in the body from its embryonic conception. Essence gives form, *Qì* gives movement, both allow life to express itself.

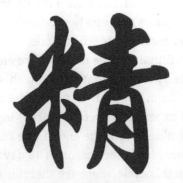

JĪNG, THE ESSENCE.

The Essence circulates through the eight Extraordinary Vessels, which form the basic energetic structure of the human body. The number eight refers us to the eight directions (front-back, right-left, top-bottom, surface-depth), to the eight principles of Oriental diagnosis (Yin or Yang, internal or external, Cold or Hot, Empty or Full), to the eight therapeutic rules of Chinese medicine (sweating-vomiting, cooling-warming, toning-dispersion, purgation-harmonization) and to many other aspects of Chinese culture, because eight is *the* lucky number par excellence. In Taoist esotericism, the energy framework is represented by a diamond with eight faces and 12 edges (i.e., 8 Extraordinary Vessels and 12 main channels), to imply that it is a precious gift from nature, our inner jewel.[4] But coming back to the cycles, it is interesting to know that *Jīng* circulates through the Extraordinary Vessels, the organs and the whole body in a cycle of seven years for women and eight for men, this difference being induced by the Yin and Yang natures.

It is therefore useful to break down the life of a human being into major cycles of Essence. Let's take the example of a woman from the point of view of Oriental medicine. From the age of 0 to 7, she is a child reaching the age of reason with a *Jīng* that makes her bones grow. From 7 to 14, she is a young girl for whom the *Jīng* will trigger menstruation at the end of this period. From 14 to 21, she is a young woman who will discover sexuality and find a companion, but the *Jīng* stops bone growth to favour reproduction. From the age of 21 to 28, she is a young mother (the *Jīng* promotes inner growth) who gives birth to her first or second child, depending on the country. Between the ages of 28 and 35, she is in the prime of life, a hardworking mother, her *Jīng* is at its peak. Between the ages of 35 and 42, in the middle of life, the *Jīng* slowly begins to decline and existential questions arise. From the age of 42 to 49, *Jīng* urges her to slow down and her body refocuses to preserve itself. From the age of 49 to 56, the *Jīng* is no longer sufficient to irrigate the uterus; this is menopause, bones become brittle and the body begins to shrink. According to classical Chinese medicine, the masterpieces of which were written a long time ago, the *Jīng* cycle stops here, because being 60 some 3000 years ago meant reaching the threshold of death.[5]

In my sessions, I always ask the person's age, because from the point of view of the *Jīng* cycles, it's very revealing to understand where they are in their life path. One day, a man came to see me with terrible back and intestinal pains. It could have been an eating disorder inflaming the intestines and causing lower back pain. But he was 48 years old, and *Kikai* (CV 6) and *Kangen* (CV 4) points were blocked and painful. The *Jīng* is to blame. By questioning him, I understood that all he cared about in life was his career, success, and money. He was at the end of his fifth Jīng cycle (40 to 48) and had not had a mid-life "crisis". In reality, there is no crisis at this age, just an intense questioning about the role of the living being and its purpose on earth. When we ignore this mid-life passage – I prefer that expression – the suffering will be there when we enter the next cycle. Years of ignoring this questioning, of not thinking about our mission as human beings, of not accepting that we are approaching death, mean that the body will somatize what the mind cannot reach. The sessions revolved around these fundamental questions, with just the hands as support, without any real technique. The day I spoke to him to die to oneself,[6] he looked at me with fear as if I were mad. But at the end of the session, a new light appeared in his eyes. He left in great silence. The next session he told me that all his symptoms had disappeared and that he wanted to follow my teachings in meditation, which he did for five years.

From the second to the third dimension

Once again, this cycle is very practical for a Shiatsu practitioner. It allows him to know where a person is in his life path and whether he is in sync with his Jīng cycle. The cycles are always represented by circles, but this habit is induced by the paper medium we use. This 2D medium is misleading and should not be relied upon. The Jīng cycle spans a lifetime, and we are also used to tracing a life on a timeline, a straight line from birth to death. This forgets that nature is not two-dimensional, but three-dimensional. If we draw lines and circles, how can we translate an endless movement? The first response of Buddhists is to say that life and death form a cycle and that this cycle must continue somewhere. This is why Buddhism sees existence as an endless cycle of life and death through the wheel of reincarnation or samsara. The Taoists, great observers of nature, took into account the three dimensions. Consequently, if a circle has an endless, linear movement, then it is because the circle changes state with each cycle, is never quite the same and is constantly evolving. It changes in width, in length and also depth. The circle thus becomes a spiral.

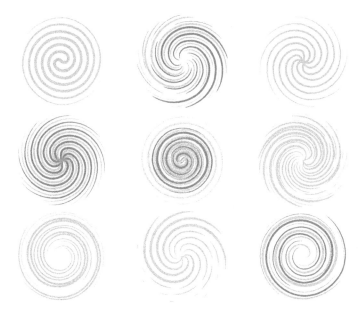

IN THIS SPIRAL, WE CAN SEE THE DOUBLE
MOVEMENT OF YIN AND YANG.

The spiral pattern is a constant in nature. Just look at the flow of water in a washbasin at home. The Coriolis force produces a spiral movement, which changes direction depending on whether you are in the northern or southern hemisphere (a Chinese person would speak of a Yin or Yang movement). The observation of trees is quite telling from this point of view. If we look closely at the main lines drawn by the bark, from the base to the branches, we can see that they twist more or less quickly depending on the species (a Chinese person would talk about the *Jīng* of the tree). Climbing plants and lianas are even more demonstrative in this respect. Climbing plants filmed in fast motion show that they always turn in the same direction to find support or hold on, following a precise spiral. As for creepers, you only have to look at their bodies to see that they are all spirals. And what about the heart of a sunflower? The spiral is everywhere in evidence as the movement of nature, as the Fibonacci sequence teaches us.[7] When it is drawn geometrically, it shows a spiral.

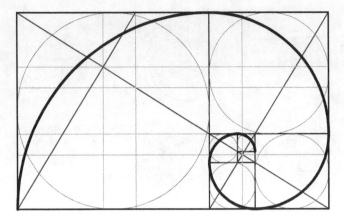

**THE REPRESENTATION OF THE FIBONACCI SEQUENCE
IMMEDIATELY GIVES A SPIRAL THAT GROWS ENDLESSLY.**

Why did nature choose the spiral? Because it answers to the Yin rising from Earth and intertwines with the Yang descending from Heaven. And the more a shape spirals, the more it answers to the principles of energy flow and therefore gains in strength. The ancients had only observation with which to deduce the principles of nature. If you observe the wind, however strong it may be, as long as it blows on a linear axis, it is possible to resist it. But as soon as it starts to turn (typhoon, tornado), nothing resists it and it tears up everything in its path. More recently, in the 20th century, DIY enthusiasts realized that a straight nail will never be as strong or as stable over time as a screw.

In the martial arts, the spiral is regularly used as a technique. In Kentjusu (warrior art of the sword), the spiral can be used in an infinite number of ways (wide or very tight) to divert the opponent's sword, particularly in the *maki otoshi* technique (き落とし).[8] In the Niten ryū school,[9] attacks are made with both swords, strongly pronouncing the vowel u with a very specific position of the tongue. Masato Matsuura Sensei[10] explained that the aim of this sound is to create a sonic spiral that disorients the partner's energy. In Qwankido,[11] Master Dong Van Sang[12] showed me that when you reach a certain level, the punches are twisted when they make contact, which gives them an incomparable – and very painful – penetrating force with much less energy than is used in Karate, for example. Finally, as you progress in Aikidō, you realize that all the techniques except for the movement of the feet are not based on circles, but on spirals that force the partner to turn and go up or down a level, the very expression of the spiral.

The spiral in Shiatsu

Shiatsu is no exception to the rule since it comes from the same cultural melting pot. In Aze Shiatsu, Shigeru Onoda understood that bodies could sometimes be so tense that basic Shiatsu pressure was not effective enough. Understanding the principle of the spiral, he developed a technique for twisting the thumbs when applying pressure. This is possible thanks to the rotation of the little fingers from the outside to the inside, which gives far greater penetration and force of pressure than most Shiatsu practitioners, while avoiding wear and tear on the joints with static pressure. Onoda Sensei justifies this technique by the fact that practitioners give a lot of Fire with their Heart and their Small Intestine, two channels located on the little finger.[13]

Apart from specific cases, most schools of Shiatsu approach the notion of *tsubos* in layers, explaining that the energy descends through three or seven layers and rises again in the same way, following the spiral forms of Yin/Yang. These spirals occur naturally when the energy is good, but when it is absent (Emptiness) or in excess (Plenitude), the practitioner's role is to tonify with one spiral or disperse with another. This spiral can be created mechanically by beginners simply by turning in the point clockwise to tonify, and counter clockwise to disperse. For the advanced practitioner, it is through intention that he or she will be able to initiate the spirals at the same time as a precise pressure without really needing to do it mechanically.

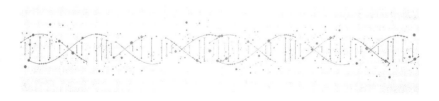

Why is the spiral so important and recurrent in nature? Because it is the most economical way of releasing the most power with the least effort. What's more, if the spiral widens or narrows, it can be wound indefinitely while respecting nature's golden ratio, which represents perfect proportion. The spiral also represents the movement of all the planets and even our suns (which are stars) around the centre of the universe. Our galaxy is shaped like a four-armed spiral and, as it is the largest we know of, we can easily deduce that this shape influences everything it contains. In fact, the Japanese have an expression that says 輪廻転生 (Rin'netenshō), which means "the soul is reborn in a spiral", clearly showing the extent to which the spiral is a principle that can be found everywhere.

Finally, the spiral is at the very heart of the life process. Water flowing through a pipe does not go straight on, but swirls in a spiral. The same goes for the blood in our blood vessels. We've recently discovered that sap from trees also rises in spirals. And if you cross a rising Yin spiral with a falling Yang spiral, you get a figure that closely resembles the two strands of DNA in our cells. Everything is in everything, as we said in Chapter 28.

Linear movement leads us to believe that life unfolds from point A to point Z. Circular movement makes us realize that every end is a new beginning, which by the way gives us hope because there is no longer a definitive end that would lead us to nothingness. But the spiral movement tells us that cycles do not repeat themselves in exactly the same way. The next circle is always a little higher or lower, a little shorter or longer than the previous one, because while life is all about movement, it is never quite the same. In this way, the practitioner understands that there are never two identical sessions, because his client is never the same from one week to the next. They have lived in between. They have experienced emotions, received a great deal of information, eaten at least 21 meals, aged a week, and their energy has travelled seven times around the 12 channels, or 21 times around the entire body. They are therefore never the same twice, just like the practitioner. This is why, although there are principles and basics, there can be no ready-made recipes. This is the difficulty and the beauty of Shiatsu: the obligation to start again each time, to question oneself, to feel rather than analyse, to let go rather than control. This is the essence of *shoshin* that we have already spoken of.

Summary

1. There is no such thing as a straight line in nature, it is a creation of the human mind; time cannot therefore be a linear movement.
2. Everything is a cycle, and cycles are numerous and affect every aspect of the world, the seasons and mankind.
3. But cycles are constantly evolving, so their representation in 2D is not correct; you have to go into 3D to realize that in reality everything that lives has a spiral movement.
4. The spiral is the most common form of Life, from the shape of our galaxy to the tiniest movement.
5. Energy moves in an upward (Yin) and/or downward (Yang) spiral.

32

A Disease Does Not Arise Spontaneously

D uring one of my trips to China, I heard a saying that went: "Good health does not augur well." Because life is a Yin/Yang movement, the body moves from one state to another, from health to illness, from one emotion to another, from one age to another. The urban myth of our societies declares that normality is good health. But between illness and good health, the point of balance cannot be one of the two, because they are extremes. It has to be somewhere in between. Perfect balance is a quest that only the masters have just about mastered; but for ordinary mortals, we regularly move from one state to the other, like a pendulum swing. That being said, while good health is not a good sign (i.e., we can only fall ill at any moment), it does mean that illness is good news because it brings the hope of recovery. In this respect, medical science is increasingly accepting the benefits of being ill from time to time. People who live a long life are not those who are never ill, but those who once or twice a year have to deal with benign illnesses with which we are all familiar (we are not, of course, talking about serious illnesses), such as the common cold, tonsillitis or even influenza. But why? Because these illnesses are constantly mutating. "Catching" one of these illnesses allows you to update your immune system and so defend yourself better. There's nothing worse than constantly blocking an aggression that comes back every year. If you do this for five or six years in a row, the next viral attack will be particularly painful. Think about the antivirus programme on your computer. If it's not updated regularly, viruses will first destroy your software and then your operating system. The idea is the same. That's why falling ill is a good sign. Each time, you adapt and get stronger.

The causes of disease

As we discussed earlier, movements are continuous and rarely sudden, except in exceptional cases such as accidents or major emotional shocks. As a general rule, it is a gradual process. This leads us to consider the reasons for illness, which the Chinese used to define as "perverse energies" (*Xié qì* 邪气). There are many explanations depending on whether you study Greco-Roman, shamanic, Oriental or any other traditional approach to medicine. Japanese *Kanpō* medicine states 因縁生起 (*in'nenshōki*), the primary meaning of which is "the occurrence of fate", in other words that "everything has a cause". According to it, these are diet, emotions, constitution, climate and old age. Chinese medicine, on the other hand, classifies causes slightly differently.

- **External causes** (*wài yīn* 外因): these are mainly climatic factors that attack the body. Chinese medicine categorizes six climatic factors: Cold, Dampness, Wind, Summer-Heat, Fire and Dryness. If they are mild and in keeping with the season, they pose no problems. But if a person ignores them, he will suffer their aggression. They then turn into perverse energy. We've all had at least one experience of a cold wet spell that quickly turns into chills, then a fever coupled with a profuse runny nose, so we understand that climates are indeed pathological causes if we don't dress accordingly. So, we're dealing with a penetration process that goes from the outside to the inside of the body.
- **Internal causes** (*nèi yīn* 内因): this can be a physiological imbalance between the organs, the cause of which could be, among other things, a poor diet or lifestyle. For example, eating fast food every day and spraying yourself with aluminium-laden deodorant is a quick and effective way of upsetting organs, particularly the liver. But there are also energy imbalances that disrupt the channels and the relationships

between them. Emotions are one of the most important internal pathological factors. The seven emotions are: joy, anger, anxiety, worry, sadness, fear and fright. Sadness, for example, will weaken the Qì of the Lung, and the person will feel tightness in the chest, a lack of energy and the desire to cry. Joy is a pleasant emotion, unless it becomes overwhelming. In this case, we fall into a kind of hysteria with uncontrollable laughter, a tendency to follow anything that is exciting, having trouble sleeping, and so on. Emotions can be subtle and slowly but surely undermine our mind. The mind is generated by the brain, which is constantly connected to the rest of the body via exchanges between the nervous and endocrine systems. As a result, it reacts to thoughts and emotions, gradually deteriorating, becoming inflamed, intoxicated and eventually completely dysfunctional.

- **Trauma**: in Chinese medicine, this category is a bit of a catch-all, including poisoning, venomous bites, accidents, epidemics, and so on. It is easy to understand that we are dealing with violent pathogenic or traumatic causes for which there is little or nothing for monitoring the onset of an illness. In these cases, it is generally necessary to react urgently and rush to the nearest hospital.

- **Lack of movement**: I'm deliberately adding this category, which is well known to masseurs, physiotherapists and other posturologists. These days, more and more people either don't move or don't move enough. We've gone from a pre-war society where people spent eight to ten hours on their feet and on the move, to a post-war society that does exactly the opposite. All our energy is taken up by brain activity; the Shén (the Spirit) is depleted without the body compensating with sufficient physical activity. The body becomes clogged (particularly the joints), excess weight becomes the norm, and muscular, tendon and bone blockages and accidents multiply. This should come as no surprise, as the body is first and foremost a locomotor system that needs to function regularly to be in good shape (compare the weight of your muscles with that of your brain and you'll quickly understand which should take priority). We therefore promote sport in all its forms. There isn't a doctor who doesn't repeat this message: "Do sport, it's good for your health." And it's true. This message didn't appear until the 1980s, before which nobody really needed it. But people can't do everything that's out there, and generally stick to one particular sport. The problem is with repetition of a sport as, for example, running wears out the knee joints, tennis the elbow and shoulder joints, and so on. There are very few all-round sports that allow you to move your whole skeleton and all your muscles without jolts or repeated mini-traumas. While we're on the subject of the absence of movement, we should also consider the immobility of the brain. By doing the same thing over and over again, the cortex no longer learns anything and loses its neuroplasticity. Once again, we get bogged down in habits, making impossible what has always been the great strength of the human being: adapting to new situations and evolving thanks to new techniques or knowledge.

- **Spiritual loss**: this last category comes from my experience as a practitioner and teacher of meditation. The loss of the meaning of life (which boils down to growing up, studying, working, and then dying) is a terrible evil today that makes life completely absurd. The break with faith or belief is another. In the absence of everyday spirituality, most of our fellow citizens have lost touch with the marvellous, with Heaven and, as a result, with their purpose. It's no coincidence that yoga, meditation, life coaching and spirituality of all kinds are so popular. Without the link that reconnects us to our original Oneness, we lose the will to live. Accumulating possessions and money is an experience that always leads to disappointment, boredom and fear (of losing). It is by no means a guarantee of happiness, quite the contrary. The absence of meaning in life leads straight to a loss of bearings, depression, drug-taking and extreme sports in order to "feel alive". But there's no need to put yourself in danger to feel alive. Reconnecting with yourself (body and mind) is more than enough. The same applies to the world of work, where employees are increasingly asked to carry out thousands of small tasks every day, without ever seeing the big picture or the satisfaction of finishing the job. It's mind-numbing and exhausting. Add to that the relentlessness of certain management or production methods and you get some magnificent burn-outs, which are almost always a combination of exhaustion, loss of meaning and harassment.[1]

Progression logic

Once we have identified the causes of the illness, it is already easier to understand that in most cases it follows a progression. Let's ask ourselves the following question: why is it that out of three friends walking together along a boulevard on a windy day, dressed in the same way, one gets a cold, another a headache and the third nothing? It only depends on the energy we have at our disposal to protect ourselves from external aggression, as if we had a suit of armour made up of several layers. External pathogenic factors must pass through these layers, the first of which is the defensive Qì (Wèi qì) that runs under the skin (according to the classics of Chinese medicine) but also all around us via the etheric body. The disease must then pass through the barrier of the epidermis and dermis, then the muscles, the nourishing Qì (Yíng qì), the Blood and the channels before affecting an organ, or worse, reaching the layer of Jīng in the Extraordinary Vessels.[2] All these layers form barriers capable of resisting and defending themselves, and the practitioner must always analyse how far the disease has penetrated. He can then support the layers that are still solid and push the problem outwards.

When it comes to internal pathogenic factors, the problem is a little different because it doesn't have to pass through the layers to reach the depths. An emotion comes from within. It can therefore sabotage the body and disrupt energy, as we see in the case of blood, bone or, worse still, marrow problems. But the idea of the treatment will be the same, to support the energetic and physical layers that are still alive and kicking the disease outwards. This is why skin reactions during treatment are a good sign. It's the Xié or the Shā[3] coming out through the pores of the skin. Trying to counteract eczema or psoriasis with cortisone cream only suffocates the disease and pushes it back inside. The symptom disappears but the cause remains untreated. We can't say it often enough: it has to come out! It's not for nothing that the sauna is recognized as being highly beneficial, as it allows you to sweat and eliminate toxins. The same applies to a technique such as Guāshā,[4] which seeks to bring up toxins through the skin.

To find out in which layer the illness has arrived, the practitioner has several tools at his disposal, starting with assessing the time that has elapsed since the onset of symptoms. The longer a problem is ignored (the famous "it'll get better tomorrow"), the deeper it becomes rooted in the body and in the deeper layers of tissue. Taking the pulse is a first-rate tool for finding out in which organ and in which layer the problem lies. Taking the pulse is an art in itself, but the basics are fairly easy to learn. On the surface we check the Yang, in the deep layer the Yin, and between the two the Blood. The observation of the tongue indicates the state of the person in the moment and it is generally on this that the practitioner bases his final energetic assessment. Of course, especially in Shiatsu, palpation is an essential means of assessing the situation. Are the tissues soft, hot, cold, tense or hard? Are the channels full, supple, tonic, or tense, empty or hard? The same thing can be done on the Source, Master or Crossing points to quickly assess the situation. Finally, there are a number of reflex zones, and those of the hara according to Masunaga are particularly appreciated for their ability to assess the situation. It is also possible to use the direct touch of organs, which is just as effective and much quicker.[5]

This vision of the disease's progression helps us to understand the layers through which it has passed, and thus to explain the many, and sometimes highly varied, symptoms that appear. This explanation is reassuring for the patient, who finds logic in what is happening to him. We often see people who say that they have pain in a particular place and have no explanation from the doctor, other than, in desperation, this little killer phrase: "there's nothing wrong with you, everything's fine", or "it's all in your head". This shouldn't be a condemnation, because it's true that sometimes it's in the head that things happen, but pain is always a signal from the nervous system informing us of a disorder in the body. It is therefore necessary to provide a physical response, even to a psychosomatic problem, even if it means doubling the treatment with psychotherapy. In this way, we make sense of what is happening to people.

Take a frozen shoulder, for example. This is a common problem, especially in women over 50. It always sets in little by little until the person can no longer move the shoulder without experiencing great pain. A *shiatsushi*, with his global vision of the body, mind, emotions and energy, can provide one or more explanations for the cause. These can be as varied as a blocked emotion following the repetition of a negative message ("you're no good, leave it to me, you're incapable", because the shoulder represents the unconscious part of our actions), a chill in the intestines (the two channels of which go over the shoulder), the after-effects of an old accident felt over time, a lack of physical exercise and movement (especially with age), a fear of starting something new, of hurting oneself, of taking risks, or even an old vaccine in the local muscles (trapezius, deltoid, levator scapulae...) that has not circulated properly. And the list goes on. By explaining what is happening, the patient is reassured and feels confident in the practitioner's ability to find a solution. The discourse in this chapter often annoys the medical profession, which is why the "German new medicine"[6] has been excluded from the legal therapeutic field and classified as quackery. Its iron laws stipulate first and foremost that all illnesses originate from a psychological shock. This is indeed rather simplistic, but that doesn't mean it's uninteresting. In Oriental medicine, we also find that breast cancer in women and testicular cancer in men appear after a major emotional shock such as the death of a child. But this is far from the only possibility.

This reminds me of an Englishman who came to see me because he was having problems getting his wife pregnant. She was in despair about having to undergo IVF (*in vitro* fertilization) and, in fact, it was she who referred him to me. I met the man in question, who was a stock market trader, always hyper-stressed and drinking a lot of beer. After asking him to stop drinking beer to lose weight,[7] I spent three months reducing his stress, improving his sleep, and working on the Kidney and Liver meridians, among other things. Nothing worked. Discovering that the husband was somewhat imperceptive, I decided to turn to psychology. I told him there wasn't much more I could do to help him, apart from a direct massage of the testicles as my master had taught me.[8] And I mimed the gestures of twisting, stretching and rubbing. As he looked at me, the man turned pale with fright and left my office in a hurry. He never came back, so I contacted his wife a month later. She replied: "He didn't tell you? I'm pregnant! I don't know what you did during the last session, but it worked straight away." So, we mustn't deny the importance of the emotional. Let's not forget that the global approach is not allopathic or homeopathic medicine, but a system that takes into account all the relationships that exist on all levels.

Once again, the question arises: why is it useful to know about the full progression of a disease? The answers are quite simple.

- First, as we have just seen, it helps to explain the symptoms, which change as the disease progresses deeper into the tissues.
- Then it helps us to understand that there are many layers, and that we can mobilize those that are holding firm in order to fight and regain energy, stimulate the body's systems and get the Blood circulating.
- Then it is possible to establish a treatment strategy and restore the person's confidence in their own self-healing abilities.
- Finally, it offers the possibility of following the internal movement of the disease as it diminishes, moves or changes form. Think of a chill that triggers the flu. If this is countered quickly enough, it will last only two or three days instead of twice as long, but above all it will evolve to change form, turn into a cold, and eventually end up as heat or cold in the nose before being completely expelled.

Prevent rather than cure

Scattered in the air, a thousand snowflakes
On blurred things, a veil of gauze
Sunny landscapes are in a haze.
It is not spring, yet I see flowers

BAI JUYI (772–846), TANG DYNASTY POET [9]

Imagine a country, with its capital, its regions, its people, its administration and its army. Now imagine that this country is not worried about the future and is only considering short-term projects. If we think about our army, the army that protects the country, if it no longer anticipates the dangers of war, then the country will be helpless in the event of aggression. It's not when the attack is launched that the weapons need to be forged; that's far too late! It needs to have developed the capacity to react immediately by regularly updating and training itself through exercises. It is even more important that it is able to reduce aggression before it develops. This is the principle of prevention. If you now see your body as the country and your immune system as the army, you will understand the importance of keeping fit, eating well and having fully functioning organs so as not to end up like poor Bai Juyi (772–846, famous in Japan as Haku Rakuten). You'll also understand that benign illnesses need to be able to visit the country from time to time, to carry out life-size exercises that are also opportunities to bring the immune system up to date with the latest strain of flu or cold. To ensure that the internal defence system's ability to react is at its best, it's up to each and every one of us to go and see a therapist at least at every change of season, to detect any imbalances before they become illnesses. But going once a month is an excellent way of preventing most common problems.

In Shiatsu, it's this ability to detect an imbalance very early on that gives us an advantage, a head start, over all the treatments in the world. In this way, the emphasis is on prevention rather than cure. Instead of waiting for physical symptoms to appear, the Shiatsu practitioner will sense the weaknesses or excesses of *Wèi qì*, *Yíng qì*, or of the Yin or Yang layer, each of which has its own energetic symptoms. Shiatsu can then intervene at the beginning of a pathogenic process and block the progression of a perverse energy in a channel. This is where the study of the antique *Shu* points mentioned in Chapter 30 comes into its own. Chinese, Thai, Vietnamese, Korean, Indian and Japanese doctors know how to spot an illness at stage 1 or 2, whereas a hospital will only see it at stage 3 or 4, when it is already well established. Traditional medicines (or ethnomedicines), some of which include Shiatsu, are therefore capable of prevention rather than cure. And that is priceless!

One of the reasons there are so many illnesses today is that few people take the time to prevent rather than cure. I have a foolproof argument for this: if you own a car, you should have it regularly inspected, repair one or two parts as the vehicle wears out, pay insurance and motorway tolls, have it serviced at the garage, fill up with petrol often, not forgetting a few gadgets that can be added for those who love their car (a new steering wheel cover, a little pine tree that smells nice, etc.). In the UK, the average annual cost of running a car is about £3800.[10] Now, how much money does a person spend per year on maintaining good health? £200, £500, £1000? How often do they go for a preventive check-up and treatment to avoid health problems? Once, twice, three times or never? Does this mean that we pay more attention and more money to a machine that is never more than a chunk of metal than to ourselves? If so, it raises questions about our sense of priorities. And frankly, when you look at it like that, four to ten Shiatsu sessions seem like a very good idea all of a sudden, and quite inexpensive at the end of the day. It is therefore essential to let a practitioner listen to every part of your body, before it plunges into pain, loss of movement or deterioration of its functions.

The body works with interrelations between all its parts and all their movements. This can be listened to and analysed very well after a few years of study. Think of what you can do just with a stethoscope to listen to the breath and the heart. Now imagine that all ten fingers are like ultra-sensitive stethoscopes, and you'll get the general idea. These movements release an energy which, as we have seen, can be broken down into several strata (or types) and different stages of progression. All you have to do is recognize these different forms of energy (this is easier to learn than you might think) to check that the inner world is all right... or not. As soon as an energy changes frequency, it means that something is changing. For good or ill? Some changes are natural (growing up, menstruation, menopause, etc.) and others are less natural and will not be pleasant to experience (reread the section on the causes of illness earlier in this chapter). These changes are detected by the practitioner's hypersensitive fingers. In fact, the energy sizzles under his fingers, stings, movements are chaotic – these are all signs that cannot be mistaken. This detection is vital, because it allows us to spot what is going wrong long before it becomes a symptom, and later, an illness. Energy variations can be regulated relatively easily as long as we work at this level, which is still energetic. Once you move into matter, it's obviously more difficult to take action, but not at all impossible. It just takes longer and is more complex. Prevention can therefore be summed up as follows: act on the roots of the energetic imbalance before it takes root in matter.

A basic question then arises: how is energy created?

Answer: with the air we breathe, the food and drink we ingest and, of course, the heritage passed down to us by our parents.

The Shiatsu practitioner intervenes at the level of energy imbalance, which is good enough, don't you think? But the individual can intervene ahead of the creation of this energy by paying attention to the way they breathe, by looking after their diet, by working on their thoughts and emotions, and by reinforcing the weaknesses from their parental heritage. As everything is in motion, it is also possible to change everything.

By the way, do you know what is the secret of Shiatsu masters (and other energy techniques) to avoid falling ill? They work on themselves every day (breathing, diet, bodywork, spirituality) to increase their energetic vibration. The higher the vibration, the less room there is for aggression of any kind to reach the body. But it's all down to personal self-discipline and a consistency of work that doesn't leave room for improvisation. So dear students and practitioners, roll up your sleeves and set an example for your patients.

Summary

1. Illness doesn't just happen; it is not bad luck, you don't just catch something. The disease has been allowed to develop through carelessness or inattention.
2. Being ill is not necessarily a bad thing. In the case of benign illnesses, it's also a way of updating our immune system.
3. When an illness enters the body, it passes through several layers, each of which provides an opportunity to block its progress and fight it.
4. Prevention is better than cure. Prevention is the great strength of Shiatsu.

33

The Body Heals Itself

I bandaged him, God healed him.

AMBROISE PARÉ (1510–1590)

Ambroise Paré, the great 16th-century surgeon and anatomist who left his mark on the history of medicine, used this phrase to explain the care he gave. This beautiful statement is important because it explains that doctors and healers of all horizons do their work, but that it is God (or Nature, Heaven, the Spirits, or whatever you want to call it instead) who alone holds the power to heal. But as the master of all healers, Jesus, said when he laid his hands on a patient: "I am the Father", so God again. Of course, Ambroise Paré's time was religious, but so are the traditional practitioners of every human culture. They all work on their spirituality. Just think of the Amazonian Indian shamans who are both healers and intercessors with spiritual entities, or all the witchdoctors of the world – they all connect to something greater than themselves. In Shiatsu, we are not cut off from this principle, except that the practitioner relies on nature and the living forces it puts into every body it has created. In the book *Shiatsu-Hō*, published in 1939, the founder of Shiatsu, Tenpeki Tamai, states at the end that it is imperative for every Shiatsu practitioner to work on meditation and spirituality. Indeed, he recommends learning and reciting the Sūtra of the Heart (般若心経, *Hannya Shingyō*),[1] one of the greatest masterpieces of Buddhism. The practitioner knows little or nothing, so he connects and makes an alliance with that which is greater than himself.

The practitioner has an obligation of means, of knowledge, of techniques and of individual quality, which he makes available to the recipient. Thanks to all this, he establishes a treatment strategy based on the pathology, on what he knows of the human body, its energies and the forces that inhabit it. He will then deploy his skills with his hands, but also with moxas, percussions and advice on health, nutrition, lifestyle, and the intensity of his presence. He will stimulate energy where it's lacking, recirculate it where it's stagnant and disperse it where it's in excess.

It's always instructive to read the biographies of the great Japanese masters. Morihei Ueshiba (1883–1969) took up martial arts in his youth, as he was weak and often ill. He went on to become one of the strongest and most energetic martial artists and founded Aikidō. He lived to be 83 years old with a strength beyond comprehension, notably by pulling up tree stumps by hand. In another field, Yukikazu Sakurazawa (alias Georges Oshawa, 1893–1966) was also of weak constitution and contracted tuberculosis as a child. Several members of his family died from it. He sought to cure himself, developed macrobiotics, which met with worldwide success, and lived to the ripe old age of 73. Haruchika Noguchi (1911–1976) was in relatively good health until he contracted diphtheria as a child and lost the ability to speak for a time. Acupuncture and herbal medicine healed him, and he developed a great energetic capacity at an early age. In 1923, the Kanto earthquake devastated Tokyo, making it impossible to sort the dead from the survivors. So, when he was just 12, he decided to send the Ki from his fingers into the ears of unconscious people. Those who were alive reacted and were taken to hospital. He became a renowned Seitai master. Reishin Kawai (1931–) was also a rather weak child and took up the martial arts to become stronger, but seriously injured his knee. Shiatsu, acupuncture and a special diet cured him. He became a tireless teacher of Aikidō and Shiatsu throughout half of the South American continent. it's a similar story with Hirokazu Kobayashi (1929–1998), who was a true whirlwind of energy and taught Aikidō and Shiatsu. Kanbun Uechi (1877–1948) was a young Okinawan who wanted to become strong because he felt weak. He left Okinawa for China to learn martial arts. He is the founder of Uechiryū Karate, a very powerful form that develops the body to be incredibly resistant and a foolproof Wèi qì. Generally speaking, all the great masters had to look deep within themselves to find the energy they needed to pursue their goals. But it's important to understand the inner workings of the energy system, as technique alone is not enough. When it comes to harnessing energy, you need to know where to find it and how to get it. This is where knowledge of interrelationships is essential.

The multitude of relationships forms the framework

Oriental medicine is not a vague science – except for those who don't study it, of course. It is an exact science within the framework of its way of thinking, its vision of the world and its dynamic concepts. If in Shiatsu we study the organs and viscera, the eight Extraordinary Vessels, the 12 principal channels and the Three Burners, we must not forget their deep trajectories, as well as the 16 channels of communication, the 12 sinew channels, the 12 divergent channels, not to mention the infinity of tiny channels and surface channels. All this makes up a dense, three-dimensional network that covers the entire body. Between all these channels, there are numerous relationships that allow the Qì to circulate throughout the body. This network is fundamental to understanding how the body recovers.

- The relationship between the organs and viscera (Zàng fǔ 脏 腑): Chinese anatomy specifies the nature of these relationships, which are sometimes very close and sometimes more distant. For example, you can't talk about the Stomach without automatically hearing the word "Spleen" as these two are so closely linked. On the other hand, the relationship between the Pericardium and the Triple Burner is much less intimate.[2] All the organs have relationships, which are not necessarily mentioned in the basic theories.
- The relationship between the Five Movements (wǔxíng 五行): as we saw earlier, these are the relationships of generating (Shēng 生) and supporting/controlling (Ke 克). But there are two others, which are the cycles of aggression (Chéng 乘) and offence (Wǔ 侮), which allow us to understand the pathogenic relationships between these five great forces of nature.
- The relationship between points on the same meridian (Tōng

jīng 通经): checking that the meridian is clear and that the points on it communicate with each other. The Chinese word literally means "to cross". This is the principle of energy circulation. In English, the term is "coalescence".[3] This work is the basis of all Shiatsu practitioners.

- The relationship between the channels of a Yin/Yang pair (*Biǎo lǐ* 表里): this is known as the surface–depth or inside–out relationship.[4] The Kidney (Yin) channel, for example, is linked to the Bladder (Yang) channel. We are again in familiar territory for all practitioners. This relationship means that one channel can be used to support the other.

- The relationship of communication and mutual aid (*Bīnkè zhǔjī* 宾客主机): in a Yin/Yang pair of channels, we can use the host-guest principle (*Bīnkè zhǔjī*), i.e., the Source point (*Yuán*) of one towards the Communication point (*Luò*) of the other. The aim of this manoeuvre is to improve the weakened channel.

- The flow relationship between opposing channels (*Zǐ wǔ liú zhù* 子午流注): on the Chinese clock, the channels are linked by opposition according to the Midday-Midnight law (*Zǐ wǔ liú zhù* translates as "channel flow"). This makes it possible not to work at night and still be able to influence the Gall Bladder channel (whose peak activity is between 11 p.m. and 1 a.m.). We can then use the Heart channel (which is its opposite between 11 a.m. and 1 p.m.) to stimulate it.

- The relationship between the channels of the same energetic layer (*Liù céng* 六层): in the principle of the Six Levels, the channels alternate as Yin-Yin, Yang-Yang. This is how the Kidney channel also relates to the Heart channel (*Shǎoyīn*), and the Small Intestine channel to the Bladder channel (*Tàiyáng*). If a Yin channel weakens, it can be supported by a Yin channel with the same level, the same energy potential.

- The relationship with the deep path of a channel (*Shēn jīng* 深经): in the 12 channels, not all their paths are accessible, only the surface path which contains the pressure points. The deep path of a channel is nevertheless very useful to know because it allows us to act on the channel or the organ. For example, the deep pathway of the lung goes around the navel, so massaging this area will unblock the channel's energy flow.

This also explains the importance of the point GV 14 (*Dà zhuī* 大椎) located under the seventh cervical vertebra, where all the Yang meridians meet and cross each other via their deep channel path.

- The relationship between points of the same therapeutic family: each point has several therapeutic effects. The families of points group them together by theme, for example the points which chase away Wind, Fire, Dampness, etc. This study is a little more advanced but necessary, and all schools of Shiatsu use at least the Source (*Yuán*), Assent (*Shu*) and Belly (*Mu*) points. There are many others, such as those which combat pathogenic factors, those that have effects on the Spirit, Heaven, Earth, Man, psycho-visceral entities and so on. Using all the points in the same family increases the desired effect.

- The communication relationship within an anatomical area (*Luójīng* 罗经): the *Luò* channels (and no longer just the points of the same name) allow the energy to irrigate an anatomical area of varying length or width. The sinew channels do the same. Knowing about them enables us to understand why one area of the body reacts the way it does, and not another, and to which organ it is linked.

- The relationship with the movement of energy (*Qì yùn* 气运): when a person is trapped in their mind, it is not useful to use channels with rising energy. This would only aggravate the symptoms. It is better to use a downward movement of energy to help them leave their thoughts behind. If a perverse energy tends to enter, it must be removed. This is why the directions of the energy are: up (*Shēng* 升), down (*Jiàng* 降), out (*Chū* 出) and in (*Rù* 入).

- The relationship with the directions (*Bā gè fāngxiàng* 八个方向): there are eight directions in total, which oppose each other two by two. The right side is opposed to the left, which is why the less painful side is usually treated, as its relationship to the opposite side helps to begin to relax and relieve the pain. The same applies to up and down, front and back, surface and depth.

- Anatomical relationships: Chinese medicine knows the human body well and has even created sinew channels (*Jījiàn jīng* 肌

腱经). The Chinese were the first in history to dissect people...
alive, to observe dynamic relationships. Anterior, posterior
and crossed muscle chains are invaluable to the practitioner
in helping to rediscover the body's natural movements. The
same applies to the joints. There are also relationships between
the curves of the spine. Relaxing the neck improves the lower
back and vice versa.

- The proximal–distal relationship (*Jìn xué yuǎn xué* 近穴远穴):
  there are many points well known to *shiatsushi* for treating
  pain locally. What is less well known is that there are also
  numerous distal points to treat an anatomical area. This
  knowledge is really useful when the pain is too severe to be
  touched. For example, for a neck problem such as a torticollis
  type: local points: BL 10, GB 20; distal points: GB 39, SI 3, TB 5,
  TB 8, BL 60. It is very useful for the practitioner to have this
  table of points nearby.

- The relationship of the Three Treasures (*Sānbǎo* 三宝): this is
  the relationship between *Shén*, *Qì* and *Jīng*. Each of these types
  of energy can help the others. When the *Qì* is depleted, the *Jīng*
  acts as a reserve and comes out at the Source points. When *Qì*
  (in this case *Zhèng qì*) and *Jīng* (or *Jīng qì*) are exhausted, as in
  cases of severe burn-out, the energy of the Spirit (*Shén qì*) will
  be the spark that starts the machine running again (hence the
  importance of meditation and spirituality).

There are other relationships, and thanks to our knowledge of Western anatomy we can add many more, but the above list already goes
a long way towards improving a person's energetic state. All these
relationships are interdependent and form, I repeat deliberately, a
web which allows organic life to exist. If one or two threads become
stagnant (let's not forget that it's all about circulation) or empty, the
rest of the weave holds firm. When you pull a thread from a carpet,
the whole carpet doesn't unravel, at least not immediately. Now
imagine a three-dimensional carpet. It's not ready to unravel at the
first blow. And this carpet is the human body.

The forces of self-healing

In Japan, they say 自然治癒 (*shi zen chi yu*): "The body heals itself."
How? Simply because of the interconnections between the relationships linking all the parts of the body, from the smallest (an atom) to
the largest (the skin), which facilitate the circulation of energy. This
continuous circulation concerns all aspects of energy: *Jīng, Qì, Shén,*
Blood and Organic Fluids. A well-placed nudge from the *shiatsushi*
can revive, increase or calm its flow, but cannot change the nature or
number of these relationships. This is what is known as "bringing the
self-healing forces into play". In other words, it's a matter of using
everything that works well in an individual to restart movement,
to put breath and energy back into the parts that are disturbed or
deficient. This is how the body heals itself. It's not the practitioner
who does this, because many of us have seen that, given a little time,
the body often gets back on track on its own, back to homeostasis. At
least in most cases. When you receive help from a practitioner, it is
not the practitioner who heals you, but rather the living forces still
intact in the human body when they are correctly reactivated. This is
a humbling experience and a reminder that the practitioner is, once
again, at the service of his fellow man and not the other way round.

When a channel is stimulated, it begins to vibrate more strongly.
The person will feel hot, cold, shivering and currents through their
limbs. The increase in its potential will either strengthen it or send
the overflow of energy to the next relationship. This overflow automatically flows into the next channel, according to the principle of
sequencing inherent in the Chinese clock. Then all the relationships
listed above will follow one after the other, layer upon layer, where
everything is connected. The energy gradually seeps in everywhere,
re-establishing communication between the major systems, layers
and different forms of energy. In this way, the *Qì* of an organ can
restore the *Qì* of the Spirit, helping us to overcome a psychological
illness, and vice versa.

But all this doesn't happen immediately. While the mind can come
up with 200 ideas a minute, the body needs time to repair itself. That's
why rest is so important, to allow the body to act and not disperse its
energy. It needs to concentrate on a single essential function: repair.
That's why sleep and the night are so important. Have you noticed

how, after a good night's sleep, you're back on top, your batteries recharged and your body ready to conquer the world? That's when everything's going well.

When we are out of balance or ill, we need a longer recovery time. But this recovery time also requires, for it to function properly, several sessions to repeat the information we are trying to communicate to it (circulation, dispersion, toning, harmonization). Energy is an information system, and it takes time and repetition to get the message across to every corner of the body. Take a muscle cell. If it's in good shape, a simple massage using kneading and pressure will do it good. Cells like to be slightly compressed to "bounce back" better, or rather to round out better, which is often their natural shape. The pressure will stimulate exchanges, cleanse toxins and encourage the mitochondria to produce energy. What's more, the nervous system makes no mistake, sending an almost instantaneous signal to the brain to relax and feel good. When the cell is in poor condition, it is tired and tense (literally: the cell stretches and becomes tense). Together with their neighbours, they tense the muscle fibres and you will find knots, tensions and cables under your fingers. Simple pressure is no longer enough to relax them; you need to work on them for longer, nourish them with water, reopen the blood and lymph circulation and, finally, send sufficient Qì to give them the vital tone they need to function. By doing this manual and energetic work, the Shiatsu practitioner re-informs the muscle in its entirety and all the cells that make it up, right down to their very core. By repeating the message sufficiently, the cells integrate the information and will tend not to repeat the error or the disturbance of which they were victims.[5] This is why it is often said that the practitioner is also a kind of silent teacher who educates the body and shows it the path to autonomy.

To thank and accompany

As we have seen, healing takes place in proportion to the presence of the disease, to the time the pathology has spent in the body. But the speed of its action is also related to the upkeep of the body and mind. On this point, *The Yellow Emperor's Classic of Medicine* is quite clear:

The wise man does not treat a declared illness:
He cures when there is no disease yet.
He does not treat an established disorder
But foresees it before it manifests itself.
This is what we need to understand:
At present, drugs are prescribed
When the disease is well established,
We treat disorders when they appear.
It's like digging a well when you're thirsty,
It's like forging weapons after declaring war![6]

Let's not forget that this text is 2500 years old, which puts our society and the way we treat ourselves into perspective. We are clearly at the opposite end of the spectrum from this statement. If the body is ready, lovingly tended to like a precious garden whose interactions we understand, then it will be strong and recover quickly. This is why the Chinese and Indians have handed down to us the human treasures of Qìgōng and Yoga. But the mind must be firm and calm at the same time, especially in the event of an aggression. If a person is distraught by illness, healing will take longer because the emotions and the mind also need to be calmed. On the other hand, if the spirit is well connected to Heaven, the person will thank the illness for having come to visit them, to help them improve, to seek answers within themselves and make progress on their path, or quite simply to remind them that they are mortal and must not think they are a god. He is in a state of nature and must follow the rules of the environment in which he lives, like all living things around him. There are no exceptions to the rule. Once again, meditation is the essential and - in my opinion - indispensable tool for dealing with illness, being grateful for it and making a peaceful return to good health.

Summary

1. The practitioner must connect to something greater than himself to allow the patient's body to recover.
2. The weave of all the energetic and physiological relationships allows the body to be solid and not to disintegrate easily.
3. The self-healing forces follow the relationships between all the body's circuits, filling in the gaps or calming the excesses.
4. Maintaining the body is vital, as is maintaining the mind. In the event of illness, support rather than fight. Give thanks rather than be afraid.

34

The Best Medicine
Is the Simplest

No one travels
Along this way but I,
This autumn evening.

BASHŌ[1]

The vision of Shiatsu, and of natural health in general, is focused on prevention rather than intervention, and on balancing the body, the emotional and psychological systems. It is an art of living full of common sense that should govern the harmony of our actions, and not a frantic race towards death and the exploitation of Mother Nature. Oriental medicine understood from the outset that it was better to pay a little attention to your health and your environment every day, rather than at the last minute when it's too late and illness and disorder have set in. As far as individual health is concerned, it all starts with observing the body's reactions. Every morning, it's a good idea to ask yourself a few questions and do a quick self-assessment: how are my muscles and skeleton, how are my intestines, what are my inner sensations, did I sleep well, am I hungry? This kind of self-diagnosis is very simple, provided you're willing to take two minutes out of your day to do it. What's two minutes in a 1440-minute day? If we don't take that little bit of time for ourselves, it's because we're not interested in our health or our well-being, and we're not trying to avoid illness. Why not...? But then it must be a conscious choice.

When we become aware of our body and our life path, choosing health becomes logical and we act accordingly.

Everyday medicine for good health could not be simpler. All you need to do is massage lightly, get your body moving, strengthen and stretch it a little, and take a few deep breaths. I often tell people who come to see me that it's not necessary to be an Olympic athlete, but to aim to be an everyday athlete. In other words, it's all about having a few healthy habits, a few small gestures for good health; it's about creating a light, no-holds-barred discipline to keep yourself in shape. Of course, diet plays a major role in this virtuous balance, as we've already discussed, as does the maintenance of the mind, emotions and spirit. I can't resist quoting one last time from *The Yellow Emperor's Classic of Medicine*, that book of wisdom which forms the basis of all Far Eastern medicine:

> *If life obeys the five vitalities*
> *Symbolized by the Five Elements*
> *The influences acting on it are*
> *Three in number: Heaven, Earth, Man.*
> *To ignore this principle*
> *Is to expose oneself to the attacks of vicious influences.*
> *This is the origin of life and the secret of longevity.*
> *It's the same as blue skies and clean air.*
> *If you obey this rule,*
> *You'll benefit from a strong Yang*
> *And harmful influences*
> *Will be unable to harm the body.*
> *In the cosmos lies the origin of the cycle of seasons*
> *Whose succession wise men faithfully follow.*
> *Respecting cosmic influences*
> *They are in constant liaison with the universe.*
> *To forget this is like obstructing*
> *The body's nine internal orifices,*[2]
> *And suppressing the function of muscles*
> *on the external plane;*
> *It's dissipating Wei (defensive) energy*
> *And, as a result, injuring one's organism*
> *And harming one's vital energy.*[3]

Not acting

To keep the body healthy, the practitioner does not always need blood, sweat and tears. Sometimes you must do - almost - nothing. This is the most important philosophical principle of ancient China: *Wú wéi* (无为), translated as "not acting". Taoism recommends listening, being present and waiting. Then life, the forces of nature, act unhindered, catalysed by the presence of the practitioner. He places his fingers and palms and listens intently to the breaths, silences and movements of the body. It is in this appearance of immobility that the Qì is freest to act as it should. Let's remember that excellent Latin maxim that doctors know well: "*primo non nocere*".[4] Shiatsu applies this principle to the letter, and often chooses to do less rather than more. And I'll say it again: "Less is more". For example, if you try to stimulate all 12 channels in one session, it won't do much good, and, if the person is already tired, it may make them feel worse. It's better to do just two or three channels well than to do too much. Think information. If you overdo it, you'll drown the main message in too much information, and the energy will no longer be able to concentrate on what's important, while the cells will no longer know what they need to learn and record to enable them to restore themselves. *Wú wéi* - which can be likened to the Indian notion of *naiskarmya*[5] - does not mean doing nothing, but rather "letting go" without wanting to control. The practitioner will seek to let events unfold, with his support and presence, but without becoming attached to his action or to the results. This is why we say that the practitioner has an obligation of means, but not of results, like all therapists everywhere on the planet.

In the great Shiatsu family, one master has pushed this principle to the end; this is Akinobu Kishi. He was a student and assistant to Tokujiro Namikoshi for ten years, then he spent another ten years studying and assisting Shizuto Masunaga. In the end, he decided to create a new branch, a kind of extension of Shiatsu called Seiki.[6]

Its principle is to act as little as possible, simply placing the fingers in certain places, then letting the energy act. When the practitioner is well connected to Heaven and Earth, the flow of energy acts with force and the recipient's body can be seen to move spontaneously to rectify itself. This is known as *katsugen undo*, a term found in Sotai and Seitai, but also in medical Qìgōng. My friend Frans Copers[7] continues this work in Europe. During an initiation course, he asked me to place my fingers in certain places on his head and let the Qì flow. To my great surprise, after about ten minutes his cervical vertebrae cracked forcefully, returning to their proper alignment on their own.

The intervention of the practitioner is therefore minimal to respect the deep nature of each individual. Indeed, what practitioner, therapist or doctor can say with ease what the person really needs? Marketers do, but not those who dedicate their lives to the health of others. We do not know the depths of every person who comes to see us, it's just impossible. The Shiatsu practitioner knows technical means and sometimes the shortest path to healing, but is this really what the person needs? It is often necessary for this path to go through many detours so that the person learns lessons, feels them in his flesh and integrates them. Sometimes suffering is an indispensable path to overcome our personal hells and to be reborn, cleansed from within. This is why no *shiatsushi* can answer the perennial question "how many sessions will it take to get better?" We must act as best we can, and then rely on what the body or unconscious mind chooses to do. This requires great humility, and the acceptance of not seeking results, of not knowing, which is far from easy. But in this process profoundly respectful of Man and Nature, there is a beauty that touches our hearts.

Beauty and simplicity

The simplicity of health lies in very few things: a good diet, a stimulating intellectual life, pleasure in being rather than in having, pleasant social relationships, a fulfilling job, friendship and love, all of which form an extremely positive whole. So, we need to avoid junk food, media mindlessness, the perpetual quest for money, harmful people, jobs that make no sense or go against our personal ethics, false friends, and destructive love affairs. Add to that a bit of sport, upkeep, meditation and laughter, and your health will be rock solid. And why is that? Because the better you feel, the higher the frequency at which you vibrate, leaving no room for imbalances. The less attached you are, the freer you feel, the less tense you are, the more you can breathe. It's all very simple, but you must want to get into this state of being present to yourself and enjoying every minute you have.

Shiatsu is an art. Like all arts, it can express a form of beauty. Of course, this beauty does not necessarily correspond to Western criteria, but to the Japanese criteria attached to the simplicity of Zen. Just as a Zen temple can be beautiful because of its clean lines, the absence of objects and furniture, and the simplicity of its tatami mats, so Shiatsu can be beautiful because of its lack of showiness and sophistication. Many practitioners try to create a whole aesthetic in their practice. But a few straw tatami mats and empty walls with a single calligraphy bring the place back to its essence: an empty space in which it will be possible to create an ephemeral work of art during the session. This simplicity is at the heart of Shiatsu and its treatment. There are not many professionals who can boast of always having their tools with them (*shiatsushi* have the advantage of always having their hands with them) and taking them out to do good around them, whatever the place or the time. This simplicity shows that, in the end, the practice can be considered an accessory. It is in the quality of being carried in the practitioner's heart, in the pure gesture represented by a simple hand placed on a body, in the relaxed mastery of breath and posture, in the silent and profound communication that Shiatsu is found.

From simplicity comes Emptiness.
From Emptiness comes beauty.
From beauty comes life.

Summary

1. With a little self-discipline, you can become an "everyday athlete" and stay in good health. Ten minutes a day is enough.
2. The Shiatsu practitioner acts as little as possible. This is the *Wú wéi* of the Taoists. He allows things to happen. He is acted upon.
3. Simplicity is at the heart of health.
4. From simplicity comes Emptiness. From Emptiness comes beauty. From beauty comes life.

About the Author

I van Bel has a long career in the world of Asian arts. Born in Toulouse in 1971, he grew up in La Rochelle where he started Aikidō at the age of 13, and also become interested in Karate (Shōtōkan from the age of 14, then Uechiryū at 25). At the age of 20, with a degree in journalism, he joined the *Institut National des Langues et Civilisations Orientales* (INALCO)[1] in Paris. There he studied Chinese for five years (writing, language but also literature, poetry, geography, economy and history of this country) and was introduced to Vietnamese, Japanese and Tibetan. In Paris, he followed an assiduous training in Aikidō, Kenjutsu and Iaido with his teacher Philippe Cocconi for 13 years. The latter pushed him to meet all the great teachers of Aikidō, whether Japanese or Western.

His many trips throughout Asia – and more specifically in China – allowed him to meet and appreciate the efficiency of Chinese medicine and of energetics, particularly acupuncture, thanks to his encounters with many practitioners, monks and doctors. Subsequently, in France, he discovered Shiatsu during an intensive Aikidō course and was initiated by François Dufour. During his eight years of apprenticeship, he had many teachers – in France and Belgium – including, primarily, Françoise Bataillon, Lucy de Mooy and Yuichi Kawada.

When he arrived in Belgium, he taught Aikidō for a few years and practised Shiatsu while continuing his training. During their visits to Europe or at his invitation, he followed several great Japanese Shiatsu masters (Onoda, Kobayashi, Ohashi, Watanabe, etc.) and began studying Chinese medicine with both Jean-Marc Weill and Raphaël Piotto. Following the inner transformations brought about by the practice of Shiatsu, he changed his martial orientation to take an interest in the Sino-Vietnamese arts (Qwankido, Qìgōng, Tàijíquán).

At the same time, he deepened the meditation practice he had discovered through the Japanese martial arts, by practising *zazen*. He also learnt mindfulness, vipassana and Kashmiri tantric meditation. Far removed from all dogma, he wondered how he could simply transmit this discipline of the mind to a Western audience.

It was a massage master in Thailand who taught him the principles of micro-meditation, a technique perfectly adapted to Westerners. He developed his meditation school in Brussels and enjoyed great success in this field, which he taught for about ten years. In 2010, still in Brussels, he created the Biloba Network, the first network in Belgium to impose selection criteria for massage and complementary health professionals. He developed two quality labels that were recognized in 2016 by the Belgian Massage Federation.

The following year, he co-founded the *École Européenne de Massage* (EEM) and became a full-time Shiatsu teacher and practitioner. In 2013, his meeting with Bernard Bouheret, a leading French teacher of therapeutic Shiatsu, proved decisive. He joined the *Union Francophone des Professionnels de Shiatsu Thérapeutique*[2] (UFPST), where he was recognized as a practitioner, then as a teacher and eventually as a member of the board of directors until 2019. In 2015, he created the website Shiatsu-therapeutique.org for the UFPST and was its editor-in-chief. He co-founded the Ryōhō Shiatsu style in 2016 with his friend Philippe Banai. The founding principle of this current of Shiatsu is not to confine oneself solely to the mechanical practice or energetic version of Shiatsu, but to learn about all its possibilities.

He states his intention thus: "If you have a fan but don't open it, you have little chance of getting any air. With each additional flap of the fan, you improve your ability to refresh yourself with less effort. So, you need to open the whole fan." Learning this comprehensive style involves anatomical study, physiology, psychology, energetics, ethics and deontology, not to mention meditation and Oriental medicine. Its intrinsic philosophy is based on the three levels of Heaven, Man and Earth. In 2018, he opened his own school, *l'École bruxelloise de Shiatsu thérapeutique*[3] (EBST), so that he could teach according to this philosophy. In 2019, he initiated the first international historical research group on Shiatsu ("History of Shiatsu" on Facebook) with the aim of finally publishing a clear and precise book on the origins of this discipline and stimulating the translation of ancient works. Finally, he founded the NGO Humanitarian Shiatsu Mission to promote Shiatsu where it matters most.

Today he continues to study all forms of Shiatsu, Oriental medicine, martial arts and meditation around the world, because there is no end to learning. He writes many articles on the internet and for print magazines, as well as devoting himself to his passion for Chinese and Japanese history and giving Shiatsu seminars wherever he can.

Glossary of Japanese Terms

Aikidō 合気道: Lit. "way of assembling the energies", martial art without competition.

Amate gata 甘手形: Position of the "soft" thumb with the pulp of the last phalanx in contact with the skin. Literally, *amate* means "sweet, sugary", but I like to translate it by homophony as the term "amiable". The kanji 形 is pronounced *gata* here, but it is known as *kata*, the form. It is the same word for a sequence in martial arts.

Anma 按摩: Lit. "calming with hands." Ancient Japanese massage with two branches: the Kōhō Anma branch of *Kanpō* medicine, and the well-being Anma practised by the blind.

Anpuku 按腹: Belly work technique in Kōhō Anma massage, which was taken up in Shiatsu.

Antei 安定: Lit. "calm, peaceful and stable, determined". This concept refers to stability, a concept that must apply to both the body and the mind.

Banbutsu ryūten 万物流転: Translates as "everything is movement", shortened from the phrase "all things are in motion through the endless circle of birth, death and rebirth". But when translated word for word we get "ten thousand, things, vicissitudes" that could be understood as "the 10,000 beings know many vicissitudes because everything is movement".

Bōshin 望診: Phase of the anamneses in Oriental diagnosis.

Bunshin 聞診: Phase of feeling in Oriental diagnosis.

Chinkon kishin 鎮魂帰神: Lit. "calming the mind." Meditative and respiratory technique.

Chōki 長跪: Upright position on the knees. Equivalent term: *ryōhiza tachi* (両膝立ち).

De-ai 出会: Lit. "meeting".

Enzan'no metsuke 遠山の目付: Lit. "to see the whole as the mountain in the distance". A way to observe globally without seeing the details.

Futon 布団: Cotton mattress that is unrolled to sleep or massage on.

Hanza 半座: Lunge or kneeling knight position. Equivalent term: *katahiza tachi* (片膝立ち), meaning "one knee standing".

Hara 腹: Belly, abdomen, in the physiological, energetic and symbolic sense. For the Japanese, it is the seat of the individual personality.

Harai or **Harae** 祓: This is the goal of the practice of *Misogi*, i.e., the purification of the mind through the work of the body.

Iaido 居合道: Way and art of drawing and cutting with a Japanese sword.

Iai goshi 居合腰: Sitting position with legs folded, but toes turned against the floor.

I shin den shin 以心伝心: Lit. "from heart to heart". Expression used to refer to the relationship between teacher and pupil in traditional Asian education.

In/Yō 陰 陽: Japanese translation of Chinese Yin/Yang principles.

Irimi 入身: Lit. "to enter into the flesh". Martial art movement which consists of entering in a straight line to hit the opponent.

Jitsu 実: State of Fullness where energy is blocked in a tissue or meridian. Opposite of the term *kyo*.

Jusha 受者: Lit. "recipient", person receiving Shiatsu.

Kanpō 漢方: Traditional Japanese medicine; translation means "Chinese medicine". Lit. "medicine of the Han", name of the second Chinese empire.

Kata 型: Sequence of movements for a specific purpose.

Keiraku 経絡: Meridian, or channel through which Ki flows. There are a very large number of meridians: Extraordinary Meridians, main meridians, communication meridians, divergent meridians, tendino-muscular meridians...

Kenbiki or **kembiki** 腱引き: Continuous rocking movement of the body.

Ki 気: A term that refers to the energy that flows through all things and connects all things.

Kime 決め: Lit. "the decision of the eye". It is the will that is allowed to shine through thanks to the power of the Spirit. In Shiatsu as in martial arts, it is the action that continues in the body while nothing moves.

Ki musubi 氣結び: Lit. "tie, bind energy".

Ki no nagare 気の流れ: Lit. "energy flow".

Kiza 跪座: Sitting position like *seiza*, but the toes are raised against the floor.

Kokoro 心: The Heart as a heart muscle, but also as the centre of the Spirit and feelings.

Koshi 言霊: Hips.

Kototama or **Kotodama** 言霊: Art of vibrating sounds in order to use their energy.

Kyo 虚: State of Emptiness when energy no longer flows through tissues or meridians. Opposed to the term *jitsu*.

Ma-ai 間合: Lit. "distance". It is a distance in space as well as in time.

Makōhō 真向法: Series of stretches for activating and cleansing the 12 main meridians and the 8 Extraordinary Meridians, to ease the circulation of Ki.

Meigen 瞑眩: This word has several meanings, but in the context of Oriental medicine, it means the side effects of taking medicinal plants. In the context of Shiatsu, it is the generally pleasant after-effects following a treatment.

Misogi 禊: Lit. "purification". Intense physical work in order to cleanse oneself from the inside.

Mitori geiko 見取り稽古: Lit. "looking at/capturing the technique". Way of saying that in the Oriental arts we must learn to observe rather than listen and analyse.

Monshin 問診: Observation phase in Oriental diagnosis.

Nigate gata 苦手形: Position of the "hard" thumb or "mother hand", on the point. The last phalanx is aligned with the others during pressure. Literally "bitter hand, not correct, worn, grated...". For 形 *gata*, see *kata*.

Seichūsen 正中線: Principle of verticality described by the martial arts and pertinent in Shiatsu. Word for word we can translate it as "correct, middle, line", i.e., the correct central line which is the way to hold one's spine.

Seika tanden 臍下丹田: Energy centre of the *hara*, located two or three fingers below the navel.

Seiki 整気: Extension of Shiatsu created by Akinobu Kishi, which could be translated as "energy adjustment" or "adjustment by energy".

Seiza 正座: Sitting position with legs folded under the buttocks, back of the foot against the floor.

Setsuchin 切診: Palpation phase in Oriental diagnosis.

Shiatsu 指圧.: Lit. "pressing with fingers." Therapeutic art using digitopressure.

Shiatsushi 指圧師: Lit. "expert/master in Shiatsu"; the officially recognized title. We do not say *shiatsuka* (but *karateka*) and even less *shiatsuki* which means absolutely nothing.

Shintō 神道: "The Way of the Gods" or "The Way of the Divine", a set of beliefs dating back to ancient Japanese history, sometimes recognized as a religion.

Shisei 姿勢: Term that determines strength in technical form and moral attitude.

Tatami 畳: Rigid piece of woven rice straw, usually 1m by 2m, which constituted the floor of traditional Japanese houses. It is also a unit of measurement equivalent to 2m². We will say of a house that it is 50 tatami mats (100 m²).

Tate hiza 立膝: Position with one leg folded under the buttocks and one leg forward.

Tenkan 転換: Movement in martial arts that consists of rotating to circumvent an attack.

Tenugui 手拭: Traditional Japanese scarf that is used for everything: tying back hair, mopping up sweat, covering the neck, and covering the head during Shiatsu.

Tsubo ツボ: Point of emergence of energy on the body or point of pressure in Shiatsu. Better known as *keiketsu* 経穴 "acupuncture point", when it is found on the meridians and sometimes outside the meridians.

Zanshin 残心: Lit. "to abandon the mind." Common meaning is more "continuous attention".

Zazen 座禅: Lit. "seated Zen." Current of meditation that awaits the arrival of enlightenment through asceticism and silence (Sōtō Zen), but also by solving insoluble puzzles or kōan (公) in Rinzai Zen.

Glossary of Chinese Terms

Biǎo lǐ 表里: Surface-depth or inside-out relationship.

Bīnkè zhǔjī 宾客主机: Host-guest. In Chinese medicine, we speak of *keqi-zhǔqi* 宾气主气, or host energy, guest energy.

Còulǐ 腠理: Lit. "tissue between the skin and the body" and "reason"; in Chinese medicine, it is the space in which *Qì* circulates.

Dān tián 丹田: A complex concept that can be translated as lower abdomen, spiritual homes or cinnabar fields.

Dào 道: The Way, the path.

Dàolù 道路: Martial sequences, known in Japanese as *kata*.

Guāshā 刮痧: Taoist technique that consists of scraping the skin using a buffalo horn or stone tool. By stimulating the skin with repeated gestures, it will expel toxins from the body, leaving red or purple traces which are sometimes impressive but never painful.

Huá Tuó jiājǐ 華佗夾脊: Huá Tuó was a renowned physician who lived between 140 and 208 CE, during the Eastern Han Dynasty. He was the first doctor to use an anaesthetic (cannabis-based) during an operation. *Jiā jí* literally means "between the spaces of the spine". It is a line with points that do not belong to the traditional meridians. Located 0.5 inch on either side of the spine, at the level of the intervertebral space, its action focuses on the root of the nerve bundles that come out of the spinal cord. This chain of points therefore has an action on the central nervous system. It is often confused with the first chain of the Bladder channel which is located at 1.5 inches from the spine.

Jīng 精: The Essence, deep energetic fluid of the body that underlies the body and gives it its shape.

Qì 气: Energy that flows through the meridians.

Qìgōng 气功: Lit. "energy work"; Qìgōng consists of series of movements and breaths aiming to activate the *Qì* in the meridians.

Shā 痧: Term that refers to acute diseases. It is found in the *Guāshā* 刮痧 technique whose meaning is "to expel disease".

Shén 神: The Spirit that dwells in the body and psyche.

Tàijíquán 太极拳: Internal martial art of Chinese origin whose purpose is to flow through long series of movements at reduced speed, in order to strengthen the body and circulate the *Qì*.

Wǔxíng 五行: Lit. the "five phases" or "five movements" (Water, Wood, Fire, Earth, Metal). These are one of the bases of Chinese thought.

Wúwéi 无为: Taoist concept which means "non-act" or "non-intention", but which does not mean to do nothing, but rather to let life do and follow the movement of nature and the order of the *Dào*.

Xiéqì 邪气: Literally means "erverse energy". This defines *Qì* when it is no longer beneficial to health, but when it is attacking organs or tissues.

Xūlǐ 虚理: Word for word "empty" and "reason"; in Chinese medicine, it refers to the "Pillar of the Void" aka "Column of Emptiness" and "Hollow Lane". It is a way to speak about the digestive tract, and it is a special line that is using different parts of a meridian.

Yang 阳: Type of energy belonging to Heaven; Its role is to circulate, defend and warm.

Yin 阴: Type of energy belonging to the Earth; Its role is to nourish, build and transform.

Notes and References

Foreword by Bill Palmer

1 La Voie du Shiatsu = The Shiatsu Way.
2 Seguin, B. & Pierrard, M. (2018) *La voie du Shiatsu* [Book and DVD]. Éditions Montparnasse.
3 Tagore, R. (1988) *Song Offerings* [trans. A. Gide (1912)]. Éditions Gallimard.
4 Ueshiba, M. (2013) *Budo: Les enseignements du fondateur de l'aïkido*. Budo Editions.
5 DE = Diplôme d'Etat = State Diploma.
6 Ecole de Shiatsu Thérapeutique = School of Therapeutic Shiatsu, Paris.

Epigraph

1 Tamaki, L. (2017) "Les techniques emprisonnent, les principes libèrent." www. leotamaki.com/2017/10/les-techniques-emprisonnent-les-principes-liberent. html

Acknowledgments

1 UFPST = Union Francophone des Praticiens de Shiatsu Thérapeutique.

Preface

1 Fall, S. (1996) *As Snowflakes Fall: Shiatsu as Spiritual Practice*. Hazelwood Publishing.
2 Tamai, T. (1939) *Shiatsu-Hō* [Shiatsu therapy]. 福永数間 Fukunaga Kazuma.
3 For all Japanese terms, refer to the Glossary.

Definition of Shiatsu

1 Ministry of Welfare (1957) *Theory and Practice of Shiatsu*. Medical Affairs Division, Medical Affairs Bureau.

Chapter 1

1 A fascia is a fibroelastic membrane that covers or envelops an anatomical structure. It is composed of connective tissue very rich in collagen fibres. They are known to be passive structures for transmitting forces generated by muscle activity or forces outside the body.
2 Myotatic reaction: the tissue contracts involuntarily when it feels attacked.
3 If you have skipped it, read the section Definition of Shiatsu at the start of the book.
4 *Huá Tuó jiājǐ*: chain of points located on either side of the spine, not to be confused with the first chain of the Bladder. For further explanation, see the Glossary of Chinese terms.

5   These are the tiny *Luò* meridians known as *Xuè luò* (血络), *Sūn luò* (孙络) and *Fú luò* (浮络).

Chapter 2

1   Iaido is the art of drawing the sword. Aikidō is the art of unifying the energy of movement with that of the opponent.
2   Shigeru Onoda, the Namikoshi Shiatsu representative in Europe and founder of Aze Shiatsu, often draws the attention of practitioners to this problem and confirms studies done in Japan which highlight the tendency to heart disorders in *shiatsushi*.

Chapter 3

1   Personal communication.

Chapter 4

1   Shiatsu was never invented to be a method of relaxation. The first Shiatsu book by Tenpeki Tamai is called *Therapeutic Shiatsu*. All subsequent works, particularly those by Namikoshi and Masunaga, all bear the word "therapy" or "therapeutic" in Japanese.
2   As it is done in Japan, with two- or three-year training of at least 2200 hours.
3   Bernard Bouheret is the founder of Sei Shiatsu, of the French Union of Therapeutic Shiatsu Professionals and author of the indispensable *Vade-Mecum – 108 Shiatsu Treatments*, published by Quintessence.

Chapter 5

1   This corresponds to the anterosuperior line of the iliac crests.

Chapter 6

1   This way of walking is called *namba* walking. In English, it is the amble walk found in bears, camels and trained horses.
2   This is the classic and polite way to ask "how are you?"
3   In meditation, this technique is called "making the mountain".

Chapter 7

1   This literally translates as "he pumps my air". The expression is used when someone is very annoying and intruding. In English we could use "to get in someone's hair" or "to get on their nerves".
2   In meditation classes, we speak of a diffuse attention that encompasses the whole body, a standby state without analysis of the mind.

Chapter 8

1   Under the rule of the Tokugawa shoguns, the Edo Era (1603–1868) offered a long period of peace to the Japanese people. Arts and crafts, like all of society, were codified by law. Anma massage was reserved for the blind because it was one of the few jobs they could do without too much difficulty.
2   Rocking is all movements aimed at calming, relaxing and disconnecting the mind by rocking the body. In Japanese this is called *kenbiki*.

Chapter 9

1   Yamamoto, S. (2000) *Barefoot Shiatsu: Japanese Art of Healing the Body Through Massage*. Japan Publications.

2   Tok Sen is an ancient massage technique developed by Buddhist monks in north-ern Thailand and Burma. It is practised using wooden instruments on which a mallet is tapped. The meridians are energized using light percussion and sound vibrations. Traditionally, this ancestral technique is only transmitted orally.

Chapter 10

1   Tagore, R. (1910) *Song Offerings*.

Chapter 11

1   In this regard, read *Shiatsu et médecine orientale*, Shizuto Masunaga, Courrier du Livre, 2017.
2   We must not forget the eight directions: forward–backward, right–left, up–down, surface–depth.

Chapter 12

1   Rimbaud, A. (2008) *Arthur Rimbaud: Complete Works*. Harper Perennial Modern Classics.
2   This is the subject of the study by Swedish-born psychologist K. Anders Ericsson. To learn more about this, read the excellent book *Outliers – The Story of Success*, by Malcolm Gladwell (2009).
3   According to the most advanced theories, it is actually our first brain. The first multicellular animals had to learn to manage digestion via a neural system long before they "thought", an action that would come a few hundred million years later. The intestinal "brain" has as many neurons as a dog's brain.
4   The four phases of Eastern diagnosis are: *monshin*, *bōshin*, *bunshin* and *setsuchin*.
5   Translator's note: in French, feeling/sensing can be translated as "sentir", which also means "to smell".
6   French-speaking Swiss writer and philosopher. In *The Journal Intime of Hen-ri-Frédéric Amiel* for 1864, his major work of... 16,867 pages.

Chapter 13

1   Arver, F. (2020) *Mes heures perdues, poésies*. Hachette Livre BNF.
2   *Book of the Way and its Virtue*, by Laozi, a Chinese classic essential to the under-standing of the Chinese mind.
3   This popular English expression originated from an 1855 poem by Robert Brown-ing entitled "Andrea del Sarto".
4   In this regard, we must look at the socio-cultural context in which we live. The Western world does not like pain. On the other hand, in Asia, a massage that does not hurt is considered null and ineffective.

Chapter 14

1   Baudelaire, C. & Tidball, J. (2016) *Les Fleurs du Mal: The Flowers of Evil*. Complete dual language edition, fully revised and updated. CreateSpace Independent Publishing Platform.
2   In Eastern medicine, the psyche is composed of five spirits that are linked to different organs. This is called a visceral-psyche.
3   For 14 years under the direction of Philippe Cocconi, Aikidō and Iaido teacher, and founder of Ryū-kempo. He is also a calligrapher.
4   Nakazono was an important figure in the worlds of Shiatsu, Aikidō and manual

therapy in general. He was notably the teacher of Michel Odoul, a famous Shiatsu author.

5   Odoul, M. (2015) *Shiatsu fondamental - Tome. 3: La philosophie*. Albin Michel.
6   Author's free haiku.

Chapter 15

1   Myamoto Musashi (1584–1645) was the greatest swordsman in Japanese history. He was the only one to perform 26 duels and come out alive. He wrote the *Go rin no sho*, the *Treaty of the Five Wheels*, an essential book on the art of sword strategy.
2   Heard during a Karate class, said by my master Takemi Takayatsu, 7th dan of Uechi ryū.
3   See www.yotsumedojo.com/shiatsu-ho.
4   Fukunaga Kazuma, aka Tenpeki Tamai, devotes an entire section to *Seishin Hoshin* 保身 (Correct Protection of the Mind) in his first book *Chikara ōyō Ryōhō*. In this section, he explains how a therapist should protect his own condition whilst helping to elevate that of his clients. Many medical studies claim that if a person lacks *Seishin*, his path in life and health will eventually be lost.
5   Odoul, M. (2015) *Shiatsu fondamental - Tome. 3: La philosophie*. Albin Michel.
6   In Japanese, the word "Sensei" used to designate the master or teacher simply means "one who was born before".
7   Emerson, R.W. (1864) *The Conduct of Life*. Ticknor and Fields.

Chapter 16

1   In writing with ideograms, a character (or kanji) is composed of one or more keys (or radicals) that add meaning to the word. In classical Chinese, a character could have a multitude of possible interpretations.
2   GAFAM: acronym for the computer giants: Google, Apple, Facebook, Amazon and Microsoft.
3   See the Bibliography at the end of this book.

Chapter 17

1   Author's free haiku.
2   Particularly in *Shiatsu et médecine orientale*, Shizuto Masunaga, Courrier du Livre, 2017.
3   I specify here that this is Shiatsu because there are many techniques to disperse *Ki* in excess, such as palpate-roll, sliding or friction found in Anma.

Chapter 18

1   Traversi, B. (2016) *Aikido - l'éducation et l'art du sabre selon Ueshiba Morihei*. Editions Circulares/du Cénacle, p.66.
2   Musashi, M. (2005) *The Book of Five Rings*. Shambhala Publications Inc.
3   de Saint-Exupéry, A. (2016) *The Little Prince*. Macmillan Collector's Library, p.82.
4   In meditation, this state is called "the empty mountain", which means great physical presence and mental Emptiness.
5   Poem by the monk Manzei, from the *Man'yōshū* (*Collection of Ten Thousand Leaves*), the oldest collection of Japanese poetry, dating from 760 CE. This collection contains 4516 poems.

Chapter 19

1 Descartes was a devout Catholic. His thoughts are a distortion of the Christian message because, as we are told, Jesus comes from a manual family (his father was a carpenter) and he himself was a healer by laying his hands on a person (Shiatsu/Reiki before our time?). Thus, hands speak long before the mind.

2 With the notable exception of alternative education of the methods of Freinet, Decroly, Steiner, Montessori and some others, where experimenting with the body makes it possible to learn more surely than by sitting on a chair without moving, which is not a healthy posture or a natural reflex, especially for children.

3 Meigen is pronounced *meiken* and refers to a symptom-enhancing effect after treatment. Not to be confused with the statue of Manneken, as the Belgian students like to say, in reference to the Manneken-Pis, a little statue peeing near the Grand-Place in Brussels.

4 Woerly, F. (1985) *L'esprit guide: entretiens avec Karlfried Graf Dürckheim*. Albin Michel.

5 Excerpt from *Poème de l'amour* by Anna de Brancovan, comtesse de Noailles.

Chapter 20

1 Author's free haiku.

2 I refer here to the explanation of Billy Ristuccia, American specialist in Anma and Shiatsu, School of Japanese Healing Arts (Sojha): see www.yotsumedojo.com

3 The *Shō* 証 kanji is divided into two interesting parts: the stem of "speech" is associated with the word "clear/straight/just". In other words, *Shō* is "that which is clearly stated". Originally, it meant "to explain, to bring reliable evidence or arguments to a superior".

4 In Chinese medicine, "Body Fluids" refers to all bodily fluids: tears, sweat, glandular secretions, mucus, clear saliva and thick saliva, but also other deeper fluids such as those that nourish the joints (synovia), fill the cavities of the skull (squamous cerebral fluid) and cleanse the body (lymph).

5 The lung is humid. The term "Water Passage" refers to the moistening function of the body, especially of the skin, which is done via the Lung, but also all the movements of ascent and descent, entry and exit of physiological fluids.

6 A "sesame seed" is an absence of sclera of round or oval shape, which forms a brown or black spot depending on its progression. This situation is annoying for the person because it opens a second path of light to the optic nerve.

7 NVC was founded by Marshall Rosenberg (1934–2015). It consists in not stigmatizing the other, but in sharing with benevolence his feelings of a given situation.

8 These same words were confirmed to me in Omiya (north of Tokyo) by Yasuhiro Irie, master of Kokodo jujutsu and Kōhō Shiatsu.

9 The sum of this knowledge has been unveiled and compiled in French by the masters Henri Plée and Fujita Saiko in two major works: *Art sublime et ultime des points vitaux* (2000) and *Art sublime et ultime des points de vie* (2009), Budo editions.

10 Yagyū Munenori (1571–1646), son of the founder of the Yagyū Shinkage school, was the first to write down and formalize this change in the use of the sword.

11 It is interesting to study belly approaches according to Iokai Shiatsu, Namikoshi Shiatsu and Ryōhō Shiatsu. For the brave, read Kiiko Matsumoto's huge *Reflections on the Sea*.

12 The apical pulse is the pulse perceived at the tip of the heart. It is also called MHR, or "maximum heart rate". It is found under the left breast in the fifth intercostal space.

Chapter 21

1 *Dao De Jing*, Chapter 11.
2 Excerpt from "L'Homme à la nature" by Louise-Victorine Ackermann (1813-1890), a French poet whose poems were shown to Victor Hugo when she was only a teenager.

Chapter 22

1 The common translation is the theory of the "Five Elements", but this is not quite right. The Chinese name *wŭxíng* indicates rather "Five Movements", as in the medieval idea of elementals, the living forces of nature.
2 Jacques Pialoux, *Le diamant chauve ou la traditions des évidences*, in the foreword to the first edition (AIBE, 1979).
3 Saotome, M. (1989) *The Principles of Aikido*. Shambhala Publications Inc.
4 The concept of Chinese Blood, with a capital letter, does not represent haemoglobin alone. It is indeed a red liquid, but also a powerful form of energy. If the heads/Yang side of a coin was Ki, its tails/Yin side would be Blood. The two are inseparable.

Chapter 23

1 In Chinese, these same characters read *xiānshēng*, a word that simply means "sir".
2 *Dao De Jing* (Book of the Way and Virtue).
3 The Heart is the home of the Spirit and the Brain its place of work. The Brain is one of the six Extraordinary Yang organs.
4 For those wishing to delve deeper into the *Yi Jīng*, I recommend the books by Cyrille Javary, a leading French sinologist and expert on the *Book of Changes* and Chinese thought.
5 The myotatic reflex is an involuntary contraction of a muscle that seeks to protect itself by tensing.

Chapter 24

1 Personal communication.
2 Issa, K. (1985) *Senteurs de pluie et de terre: Haïkus* [trans. M. Kemmoku]. Editions Picquier.
3 Diseases of the soul are a particular dimension of pathologies. Some people come and say that they don't know what they're doing on Earth, that their body doesn't fit, that they want to leave quickly and return to where they came from, which is not in this dimension.

Chapter 25

1 Interview with Morihei Ueshiba and Kisshomaru Ueshiba. In the book named *Aikido, Tokyo, Kowado*, 1957. Later translated into English by Stanley Pranin.
2 It is amusing to draw an analogy between Karate and Shiatsu, since the translation of the name "karate" means "the empty hand" and by extension "the hand without intention", in other words exactly as for the Shiatsu practitioner.
3 Seiki Soho was created by Kishi Akinobu (1949-2012), who taught Namikoshi Shiatsu and then Iokai Shiatsu for 30 years. He eventually stopped following preconceived ideas and patterns and let Ki express itself spontaneously.
4 In meditation, a distinction is made between the spirit (the action of the mind, which in psychoanalysis is similar to consciousness) and the conscience (closer to the soul, which in psychoanalysis is similar to the unconscious).

5   To find out more about the collective unconscious, read the work of the psycho-analyst Jung.
6   The zone where collective thought exists was called the "noosphere" by Édouard le Roy, a term successfully taken up by Vladimir Vernadsky and Pierre Teilhard de Chardin in his cosmogenesis.
7   This phenomenon is very well detailed in the lexicon of *What Your Aches and Pains Are Telling You: Cries of the Body, Messages from the Soul*, by Michel Odoul (Healing Art Press, 2018).
8   On this subject, read *Gut: The Inside Story of Our Body's Most Underrated Organ*, by Giulia Enders (Scribe, 2015).

Chapter 26
1   Issa, K. (1992) *Haiku*. Verdier.
2   I use the words of Claude Larre and Elisabeth Rochat de la Vallée in *Essence Spirit Blood and Qi* (Monkey Press, 1999).
3   The heart beats 70 times a minute, 4200 times an hour and 100,000 times a day. That's how vital it is.
4   Notably at the Faculty of Medicine in Louvain-la-Neuve, during the congress of the *Natural Health Institute* in 2017. Theme: "The human microbiome: the stomach-liver-small intestine relationship, as seen through the eyes of osteopathy and Chinese medicine".
5   Suzuki, S. (2006) *Zen Mind, Beginner's Mind*. Shambhala. (Shunryū Suzuki (1904–1971) was one of the great Zen masters of the 20th century.)
6   Read *The Power of Now* by Eckhart Tolle (Yellow Kite, 2001).
7   *The Fruits of the Earth* by André Gide (Vintage Classics, 2002), winner of the Nobel Prize for Literature.
8   Oxytocin is the love hormone.
9   Markedly in Romania under the dictator Ceausescu, and in China.
10 In *Zen Mind, Beginners Mind*, by S. Suzuki (Weatherhill, 1970).
11 "Shoshin, l'esprit du débutant", www.leotamaki.com/2015/08/shoshin-l-esprit-du-debutant.html

Chapter 27
1   Hugo, V. (2002) *Les contemplations*. Classiques – Le livre de poche.

Explanation of the Philosophical Principles of the Shiatsu Way
1   Rabelais, F. (1994) *Gargantua*. NRF.

Chapter 28
1   Author's free haiku.
2   According to the Big Bang scientific model, the primordial soup is a state of matter made up of gluons, quarks, photons and electrons.
3   "The Ten Thousand Beings" is a Taoist expression meaning "the totality of life." The number *wan* (10,000) means "that which is countless".
4   The various forms of reflexology are now very well accepted in hospitals.
5   Remarks by Serge Augier, a leading Taoism specialist, in an interview by *Shiatsu-France.com* published on 16/10/2019. www.shiatsu-france.com/article-entretien-avec-serge-augier.html
6   This is not what the teachings of Chinese medicine say: they put pharmacopoeia as the first principle, then needles and lastly the manual arts. But some Taoist

writings reverse this classification by putting in the foreground the arts without touching, then with touching, the needles, and finally the pharmacopoeia. This reversal of point of view is called "Earth to Heaven and Heaven to Earth".

7   In fact, the ancestor of Shiatsu, Kōhō Anma, had already been making full use of all the principles and channels of *Kanpō* medicine for centuries. Shizuto Masunaga simply updated what had long existed, adding his own personal touch: channel extensions.

Chapter 29

1   To go further on this subject, I, once again, refer the reader to Javary, C. (1991) "De la santé au salut", *La Revue Française de Yoga 3*, 43–56.

2   In 2015, in France, pesticides were recognized as a cause of Parkinson's disease and declared an "occupational disease" among farmers.

3   *Report of Partial Findings from the National Toxicology Program: Carcinogenesis Studies of Cell Phone Radiofrequency Radiation in Hsd: Sprague. Dawley® SD rats (Whole Body Exposures)*, 19/05/2016. www.biorxiv.org/content/biorxiv/early/2016/05/26/055699.full.pdf

4   For purists, I should point out that Oriental medicine does not like excessive perspiration, which drains the body of its Organic Liquids and dries out the tendons and ligaments. This is known as "thieving" perspiration, from which it is difficult to recover.

5   In this regard, read the excellent thematic books, of each emotion, of the Zen master Thich Nhat Hanh. See Bibliography at the end of this book.

6   There is no shortage of examples of self-destruction in the history of mankind: the inhabitants of Easter Island, the Anasazi, the Olmec, the Maya, and so on.

7   "Pourquoi gouverner si ce n'est pas pour faire le bonheur?", interview with Sabine Verhest, *LaLibre*, 08/06/2015. www.lalibre.be/international/2015/06/07/pourquoi-gouverner-si-ce-nest-pas-pour-faire-le-bonheur-LN76NIQ7AFCQFDBN3QXH6W43TQ

Chapter 30

1   For a more detailed translation, see the Glossary of Japanese terms at the end of the book.

2   This is not quite true – these same "wild" species are bred and released to hunt them better. But the result is the same: overpopulation of a species without natural regulation by predators.

3   *Dao De Jing.*

4   For example, www.dailymotion.com/video/x4ury3e

5   Ti, H. (1999) *Nei Tching Sou Wen*, Chapter 1 [trans. J.-A. Lavier]. Pardès.

6   Li Po, or Li Bai, or Li Tai Po, or Li Tai Bai (643–706) was one of the greatest poets of the Tang Dynasty period.

7   Huang-Ti (1990) *Neijing Suwen*. [trans. J.-A. Lavier]. Éditions Prades, p.22.

8   The term "antique *Shu*" (or *Yu* in Japanese) distinguishes them from the *Shu* of the back (*Bei shu*). "Antique" indicates that these are very old points in the genesis of Chinese medicine, probably among the first to be established as a therapeutic system.

9   Odoul, M. (2015) *Shiatsu fondamental – Tome. 3: La philosophie*. Albin Michel.

10   Jean-Marc Weill is a teacher of Shiatsu, sophrology and Oriental medicine. He teaches all over the world.

Chapter 31

1　The *ensō* (円相 "circle" in Japanese) is the symbol of Emptiness and completion in Zen Buddhism. It comes from the Chinese Taoist concept of *wú* (Emptiness), via Chinese *Chán* Buddhism and then Korean *Son* Buddhism.

2　The word "circadian" comes from the Latin *circa* and *dies*, the circle and the day, one complete revolution of the Earth around the Sun.

3　*Huǒ ming mén* 火命门 is one of the most powerful concepts in Taoist body alchemy. Located 4 inches behind *Ming men* 命门 point (GV 4) or 4 inches from the surface of the *hara*, it represents the mysterious heart of energy production, but also the storeroom of this same energy. It is the place where the energy of the ancestors mixes with the daily energy of the channels. This place is like an inner fire that transforms *Jīng* into *Qì* and excess *Qì* into *Jīng*. This is why we speak of *Huǒ ming mén* both as the primordial spark that gives life, but also as being the source of energetic movement since it intervenes via *Yuán qi* in all the phases of *Qì* transformation (*Kōng qì, Gǔ qì, Zheng qì, Yíng qì, Wei qì*, etc.). At this level of complexity and interaction, we can speak of a Fire of Destiny burning within us.

4　See Jacques Pialoux, *Le Diamant chauve* in the Bibliography.

5　In many countries of the developing world, this is still often the average limit. I lived in Malawi, in south-east Africa, and being 60 is already old age, close to death.

6　Using the Hollow Lane aka Column of Emptiness, or *Xūlǐ*.

7　Leonardo Fibonacci (1175–1240) proved that a sequence could be neither geometric nor arithmetic. He added the first two terms (0 and 1) to give a result, which was then added to the previous term, giving 0, 1, 1, 2, 3, 5, 8, 13, 21, and so on.

8　*Maki* means "to roll up", and *otoshi* "to cut down". The word *maki* can be found, for example, in *maki sushi*, which refers to sushi rolled in seaweed.

9　Niten ryū, or "school of the two skies". This is the two-sword style developed by the famous Myamoto Musashi (1584–1645), whose major work is the *Go rin no Shō* or Treatise of the Five Rings, which reminds us of the Five Elements in the form of circular movements.

10　Masato Matsuura is a master of Nō theatre and Kenjutsu who teaches in Paris and Brussels.

11　Qwankido is a Sino-Vietnamese martial art founded by Pham Xuân Tong, halfway between southern Shaolin Kungfu and Vietnamese Vietvôdao.

12　Dong Van Sang is a Qwankido master and head of the Red Dragon school.

13　In martial arts, the little finger is nicknamed "the strong finger", because once it is closed, it is very difficult to get out of a grip. Especially if it is partially loose according to the *go-ju* principle: tough and supple at the same time.

Chapter 32

1　In this regard, read Johann Chapoutot's *Free to Obey: How the Nazis Invented Modern Management* (Gallimard, 2020), which explains very well how our current management methods were initiated by the Hitler regime.

2　For the purists, my statement here is broader than the four layers of Chinese medicine which are used to study pathological pictures and which are, in order: the protective *Qì*, the *Qì*, the nourishing *Qì* and the Blood.

3　*Xié*: perverse energy. *Shā*: acute illness. See explanations in the Glossary of Chinese terms.

4　See Glossary of Chinese terms.

5   In Ryōhō Shiatsu, we learn a technique that can diagnose the abdomen in less than a minute. This technique comes from the Kōhō Anma.

6   The "German New Medicine" was founded by Ryke Geerd Hamer (1935–2017).

7   A big belly on a person who spends his time sitting keeps excessive heat on the testicles. This is one of the causes of male sterility.

8   True story.

9   Florence, H.-S. (1995) "Maladie et poésie sous les Tang." *Études chinoises* 14, 1, 61.

10   See www.nimblefins.co.uk/cheap-car-insurance/average-cost-run-car-uk

Chapter 33

1   This is the shortest but most important text of the Prajnāpāramitā teaching. Written between the 1st and 6th centuries CE, it teaches Emptiness (*śūnyatā* in Sanskrit) of all things and phenomena, which does not mean their non-existence, but their absence of substantial, fixed and permanent character.

2   According to Soulié de Morant, there is a relationship between the sympathetic and parasympathetic nervous systems.

3   In biology, the term "coalescence" means the normal or pathological joining together of two neighbouring tissues or organs. In Oriental medicine, the term is used to describe the connecting through communication. The acupuncturist uses this, but even more so the *shiatsushi* who follows the path of the meridians.

4   See the Glossary of Chinese terms at the end of this book.

5   We could also talk about messenger RNA, which informs the DNA code. Thanks to epigenetics, we know that every action, every feeling, every piece of information is encoded every 24 hours in sexual cells, and every two hours in neuronal cells.

6   Ti, H. (1999) *Nei Tching Sou Wen*, Chapter 2 [trans. J.-A. Lavier]. Pardès.

Chapter 34

1   Bashō, M. (2021) *L'Intégrale des haikus*. Points.

2   Just a reminder: the nine orifices are the two eyes, the two nostrils, the two ears, the mouth, the anus, the sex, plus one that has been closed: the navel.

3   Ti, H. (1999) *Nei Tching Sou Wen*, Chapter 3 [trans. J.-A. Lavier]. Pardès.

4   Translation: "First, do no harm."

5   *Naiskarmya* literally means "state of absence of all karmas or rituals and actions".

6   Kishi Sensei went through a severe depression, and hell, but inspired by Shintoism, he recovered. From this experience, which profoundly transformed him, Seiki was born.

7   A pioneer of Shiatsu in Belgium, founder of the Belgian Shiatsu Federation, then president of the European Shiatsu Federation, he was one of the closest disciples of Kishi Sensei.

About the Author

1   National Institute of Oriental Languages and Civilizations, the equivalent of SOAS University in London.

2   Francophone Union of Therapeutic Shiatsu Practitioners.

3   Brussels School of Therapeutic Shiatsu.

Bibliography

Attar, F. & Huart, P. (1999) *Shiatsu et arts martiaux [Shiatsu and Martial Arts]*. Budo editions.

Beresford-Cooke, C. (2017) *Shiatsu: théorie et pratique [Shiatsu: Theory and Practice]*. Maloine.

Bouheret, B. (2006) *Shiatsu familial [Family Shiatsu]*. Quintessence.

Bouheret, B. (2012) *Vade-mecum de Shiatsu thérapeutique [Therapeutic Shiatsu Handbook]*. Quintessence.

Copers, F. (2019) *Sei-Ki – The Practice of Seiki – Life in Resonance*. editions Seikisoho.be.

Enders, G. (2017) *Gut – The Inside Story of Our Body's Most Under-Rated Organ*. Scribe UK.

Gleason, W. (2009) *Aikido and Words of Power: The Sacred Sounds of Kototama*. Destiny Books.

Granet, M. (2013) *Chinese Civilization (The History of Civilization)*, 1st edition. Routledge.

Huard, P., Ohya, Z. & Wong, M. (1977) *La médecine japonaise – Des origines à nos jours [Japanese Medicine – From the Beginning to the Present Day]*. éditions Dacosta.

Javary Cyrille, J.-D. (2002) *Yi Jing: le livre des changements [Yi Jing: The Book of Changes]*. Albin Michel.

Javary Cyrille, J.-D. (2012) *Les trois sagesses chinoises [The Three Chinese Pillars]*. Albin Michel.

Jung, C.G. (2013) *The Search for Roots: C. G. Jung and the Tradition of Gnosis*. Gnosis Archive Books.

Kishi, A. & Whieldon, A. (2011) *Sei-Ki: Life in Resonance – The Secret Art of Shiatsu*. Singing Dragon.

Laozi (1999) *Tao Te Ching: An Illustrated Journey* [trans. Stephen Mitchell]. Frances Lincoln editions.

Larre, C. & Rochat de la Vallée, E. (1995) *Rooted in Spirit: Heart of Chinese Medicine*. Barrytown/Station Hill Press, Inc.

Lavier, J.-A. (1988) *Médecine chinoise, médecine totale [Chinese Medicine, Complete Medicine]*. Grasset.

Ligot, H. (2017) *Le grand livre du shiatsu et du do in [The Big Book of Shiatsu and Do-in]*. Leduc.

Maciocia, G. (2015) *The Foundations of Chinese Medicine: A Comprehensive Text*. Churchill Livingstone.

Maciocia, G. (2021) *The Practice of Chinese Medicine: The Treatment of Diseases with Acupuncture and Chinese Herbs*. Churchill Livingstone.

Marié, É. (Dr) (2008) *Précis de médecine chinoise [Summary of Chinese Medicine]*. Dangles.

Masunaga, S. (1977) *Zen Shiatsu: How to Harmonize Yin and Yang for Better Health*. Japan Publications Inc.

Matsumoto, K. (1993) *Hara: Reflections on the Sea*. Churchill Livingstone.

Morihei, U. & Takahashi, H. (2013) *The Heart of Aikido: The Philosophy Of Takemusu Aiki*. Kodansha America, Inc.

Musashi, M. (2005) *The Book of Five Rings: A Classic Text on the Japanese Way of the Sword*. Shambhala Publications Inc.

Namikoshi, T. (1995) *Shiatsu: Japanese Finger Pressure Therapy*. Japan Publications Inc.

Ni Maoshing (1995) *The Yellow Emperor's Classic of Medicine: A New Translation of the Neijing Suwen with Commentary*. Shambala Publications Inc.

Odoul, M. (2014/2015) *Shiatsu fundamental [Essential Shiatsu]*, Vol. 1 to 3. Albin Michel.

Odoul, M. (2018) *What Your Aches and Pains Are Telling You: Cries of the Body, Messages from the Soul*. Healing Arts Press.

Ohashi, W. (1991) *Reading the Body: Ohashi's Book of Oriental Diagnosis*. Penguin.

Pialoux, J. (2002) *Le diamant chauve ou la tradition des évidences [The Bald Diamond or the Tradition of Evidence]*. éditions Cornelius Celsus.

Rappenecker, W. & Kockrick, M. (2008) *Atlas of Shiatsu: the Meridians of Zen Shiatsu*. Churchill Livingstone.

Rofidal, J. (1983) *Do-in: The Philosophy*. HarperCollins Distribution Services.

Staemler, B. (2009) *Shinkon Kishin: Mediated Spirit Possession in Japanese New Religions*. LIT Verlag Münster.

Suzuki, S. (2005) *Zen Mind, Beginner's Mind*. Shambhala Publications Inc.

Tamura, N. (2003) *Étiquette et transmission [Etiquette and Transmission]*. Budo éditions.

Teilhard de Chardin, P. (1984) *Activation of Energy*. Harcourt.

Thich Nhat, H. (2001) *Anger: Buddhist Wisdom for Cooling the Flames*. Rider.

Thich Nhat, H. (2023) *Fear: Essential Wisdom for Getting through the Storm*. Rider.

Wilhelm, R. (1992) *The I Ching or Book of Changes*. Princeton University Press.

Notes to Meditate

....
....
....
....
....
....
....
....
....
....
....
....
....
....
....
....
....

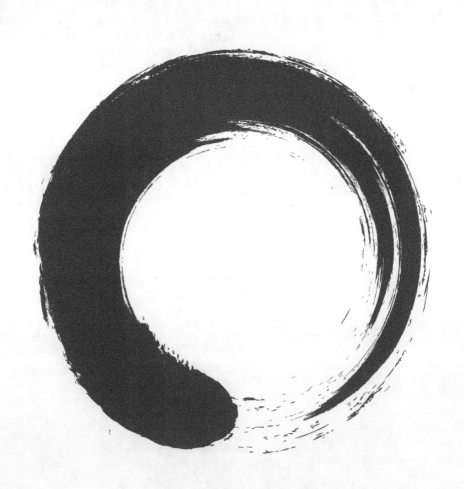